Barcode in Back

D0629425

Transitioning Exceptional Children and Youth into the Community: Research and Practice

THE CHILD & YOUTH SERVICES SERIES:

EDITOR-IN-CHIEF

JEROME BEKER, *Director and Professor, Center for Youth Development and Research, University of Minnesota*

Transitioning Exceptional Children and Youth into the Community: Research and Practice

Ennio Cipani
Guest Editor

Child & Youth Services
Volume 10, Number 2

The Haworth Press
New York

Transitioning Exceptional Children and Youth into the Community: Research and Practice has also been published as *Child & Youth Services*, Volume 10, Number 2 1988.

The Haworth Press, Inc., 12 West 32 Street, New York, NY 10001
EUROSPAN/Haworth, 3 Henrietta Street, London WC2E 8LU England

LIBRARY OF CONGRESS
Library of Congress Cataloging-in-Publication Data

Transitioning exceptional children and youth into the community : research and practice / Ennio Cipani, editor.
     p. cm.
     ". . . has also been published as Child & youth services, volume 10, number 2 1988" – T.p. verso.
     Includes bibliographical references and index.
     Contents: Historical and philosophical issues in normalization of handicapped individuals / Pat Kearly – Measurement of adaptive behavior / Howard G. Cohen – Functional skills and behavioral technology / Ennio Cipani – Teaching and training relevant community skills to mentally retarded persons / Johnny L. Matson – Research and practice in three areas of social competence / Ennio Cipani – Leisure and recreation of exceptional children / Sherwood B. Chorost – Research and trends in employment of adolescents with handicaps / John S. Trach, Frank R. Rusch.
     ISBN 0-86656-733-X
     1. Mentally handicapped children – Rehabilitation – United States. 2. Exceptional children – Rehabilitation – United States. 3. Mentally handicapped children – Education – United States. 4. Exceptional children – Education – United States. 5. Socialization. I. Cipani, Ennio.
HV894.T73   1988
362.3'83 – dc19
                                                  88-852
                                                    CIP

Transitioning Exceptional Children and Youth into the Community: Research and Practice

CONTENTS

ABOUT THE EDITOR

Ennio Cipani, PhD, is Associate Professor of special education at the School of Education, University of the Pacific in Stockton, California. He is also Program Coordinator for the Severely Handicapped Teaching Credential Program, and a licensed psychologist in California. Dr. Cipani has published over 50 articles, chapters, and language instruction materials in the areas of special education and behavior modification.

Foreword

The cultural, political, and social forces of the 1960s and 1970s have brought the American people much closer to a pluralistic society than ever before. Landmark legislation, at both the state and national levels, has enabled people with handicaps to have the opportunity, more than ever before, to reach their potential. I am proud to have sponsored legislation in California that has made possible the education of children with handicaps as well as legislation designed to produce a coordinated continuum of services for children, adolescents, and adults with handicaps.

Legislation alone cannot, however, be the sole answer. Rather, it sets the occasion for the efforts of personnel in the field to pursue the task of developing services, materials, and systems that allow people with handicaps the opportunity to learn to adapt to the mainstream of society, as we adapt to their individual differences.

This volume serves to provide the reader with some of the technological advances that have been made to accompany the social changes enacted over the years. It is astounding to encounter the changes in the instructional and educational environments that have occurred as a function of researchers asking and answering basic questions about the potential and capability of people with handicaps. Thanks to the development of such a technology, these individuals are more capable of integrating into the mainstream of society. They have learned skills previously not entertained as in the realm of possibility for handicapped people; as a result, they have changed our conception of their full potential.

These articles provide personnel in the field with a resource of such technological advancements and serve as a tribute to man's willingness to help those less fortunate, as well as our spirit of advancing the quality of life for all. As an advocate for people with handicaps, I welcome these developments in habilitative programming to enhance the quality of their lives and of ours.

Alan Short
Attorney & Former State Senator
California

Preface

The dynamic process of normalizing and mainstreaming exceptional children and youth comes alive in the chapters of this volume. Ennio Cipani has brought together a nicely integrated series of writings whose authors articulate the functional components in the technology of behavior change in less controlled environments which, in turn, provide a built-in method for evaluation.

Patt Kearly describes some of the legislation and litigation of the past decade or so reflecting emerging social concerns about opportunities for learning — or the lack thereof — among handicapped youth, particularly those in institutional settings. With new emphasis on mainstreaming and the normalizing process, there was a sort of head-in-the-sand hope that placing distressed youth in regular settings with regular kids would somehow have a positive "guilt-by-association" effect on their growth and development. In fact, the conventional wisdom at the time among practicing behaviorists was that the newly acquired behaviors — if acquired at all — would come under the control of reinforcers already occurring in the natural environment; they never did address the issue of why this "natural community of reinforcers" wasn't effective in the first place.

And of the kids who couldn't make it, one has to wonder whether that was because they deviated from average on norm-referenced testing or whether the natural environment was not responsive to their functional skill deficits. Mainstreaming meant implementing a normalization process. The effect, however, was frequently to place kids who couldn't make it back into normal surroundings with a few special effects thrown in; what they really needed still wasn't available, as we already knew. Kearly says it even better: "Opportunities for interaction are a necessary but not sufficient condition for acquiring social and personal competence."

The least restrictive environment embodied in P.L. 94-142 said the same thing in a different way, but it also mandated a formal planning process for change, the provision of opportunities for change, and accountability for end results. What was needed was a technology that would make normal patterns of behavior available to deficient children. That required some rethinking of our concepts about normal behavior, as in, what's normal? Under what conditions? And, how do we know?

And here is where this volume is exciting reading, for it traces the reshaping, or at least rethinking, of traditional developmental theories of childhood and the nature and parameters of the growth process. We already had the IQ as the standard measure of all things competent — intellectual, social, and otherwise. Given a deficient IQ — subscale or otherwise — there was presumed deficiency everywhere in the child's capabilities and development. Back to the warehouse with you!

Traditional developmental theories persuaded us that there are ages and stages through which we all must progress — stay in line, please, and there is no leap-frogging of skills, thank you — and that there are critical periods during which certain learning must occur for good intellectual and emotional growth, to boot. The result was that children were compared to these norms, which somehow sounds a little vulgar, instead of their behaviors (read: competency skills) being measured against some criterion having to do with what it was we wanted them to be able to do.

Happily, evolving behavioral technologies grounded in solid research and society's demand to empty the warehouses came together and began a minuet of mutual enhancement that continues to this day. Social, economic, and other forces as described in Howard Cohen's chapter brought the notion of adaptive behavior out of hiding as a hypothetical construct and put it to work quantifying behavioral standards of competence. We now had a concept for functionally analyzing behaviors that could be grouped according to certain commonalities and against which individual performance could be measured. Hence, we graduated ourselves from norm-referenced to criterion-referenced measures of performance, specified the behaviors we were interested in, broke them down into their component parts, and said, hey, if we can do this with toilet training, for instance, how about conversational skills, or how to apply for a job, or how to assert one's personal style!

Cohen describes the current trends in research-grounded adaptive behavior measurement all the way from socioecological to direct observational approaches, and much more. What we see happening is the development of a functional skills model of habilitation for deficient youth that contrasts with the more traditional developmental model, and that uses behavioral technology to achieve the habilitation, or skill acquisition goal, that we had in mind all the time, except now the task is conceptualized in a way that suggests intervention strategies with built-in evaluation potential.

Cipani neatly describes the behavioral model as he takes us through the what and how of training, drawing on empirical studies using strategies of chaining and shaping, among other procedures. The article provides us as well with a "top-down" model for diagnosing skill deficits, strategies for intervention, and how to adapt the training environment so that generalization is most likely to occur.

The functional analysis of behavior being what it is, its followers could not do other than analyze behavioral deficits into their smallest functional parts, seek commonalities across behaviors, and then classify accordingly. Thus, a technology utilizing the functional analysis of whole environments and methods to train people to survive and even to thrive in them is made possible. And so the remaining chapters do just that. Johnny Matson reviews the literature on self-care and other "community" skills, describing how the emphasis on community living and mainstream integration highlighted the adaptive behaviors required for survival there and the need for more sophisticated social competencies. He anticipates the feedback loop fine-tuning capability of adaptive behavior technologies.

Cipani then reviews the literature on social competence and the development of a behavior technology for training skills in conversation, interviewing, and social assertion. Enormous strides have been made in developing a technology to teach these complex social skills, although there is still much to be done. For example, Cipani discusses the need to develop a better technology for training conversational skills, and the need for better validation of training in such problematic behaviors as socially inappropriate language. The training model comprised of instruction, modeling, and behavioral rehearsal has held up well in numerous applications, but its power to train behaviors that will generalize to the natural setting needs further testing across a wider range of environmental settings and subject populations.

Sherwood Chorost discusses the importance of the skilled use of leisure time and recreation for the development of self-esteem and a sense of relatedness with the social environment. Moreover, he relates competence in recreational and leisure skills to the value that normalizing experiences have in counteracting the conditions which may support dysfunctional behavior, i.e., the concept of—guess what—the least restrictive environment.

John Trach and Frank Rusch describe research in the acquisition of employment skills for youth who heretofore were considered simply not good candidates for job skills training. They make a very potent case for integrating school curricula with the community-based delivery system of which it is a part, proposing an 8-step sequence for employment preparation that includes the community, the school, the job, the parents, and the student.

And so we come full circle: the principle of normalization, the concept of least restrictive environment, and the practice of transitioning exceptional youth to the mainstream of community life have compelled us to stretch our notions about adaptive behavior. Emerging and powerful technologies of behavior change have helped us to conceptualize deficiencies as matters of functional skill acquisition and to see how these skills could be trained in youth previously thought to have reached their developmental limits. The more research and clinical practice experience we gain with diagnostic and intervention strategies about how to train specific skills in social and personal competence, the more opportunity we see to nurture new domains of competence that are potentially susceptible to behavioral technologies. It's a question of asking the right question, isn't it?

To extend this thinking further, one needs to ask whether the social environment does not also undergo change. For example, how are the children in the classroom affected by their learning to reinforce their handicapped peer for his or her new achievements? What is the cumulative effect of increased tolerance for exceptional behavior on the social environment and on the thrust of professional technology? And so as our youth acquire more skills, increased opportunities become available for exceptional youth to generate the positive reinforcers that are available in the normalization experience. This process of constructive feedback from the application of behavioral technologies grounded in solid research and practice applied to ever-widening domains of personal and social competence is a dynamic one, and its vigor is well expressed in this volume.

Buell E. Goocher
Executive Director
Boys and Girls Mental Health Centers
El Cajon, California

Acknowledgement

The editor wishes to express sincere appreciation and gratitude to Cindy First, Department of Special Education, University of the Pacific, for her careful editing and comments on the manuscript.

SECTION I:
OVERVIEW

Historical and Philosophical Issues in Normalization of Handicapped Individuals

Patt Kearly

ABSTRACT. The treatment of handicapped individuals within our society has significantly changed over different historical periods. This chapter provides a summary of seven distinct eras reflecting the philosophical perspectives which have influenced past practice. The concept of normalization, as an underlying principle, is described and arguments within the field related to the application of a behavioral technology are presented. Implications for present practice are discussed with particular attention to legal and ethical considerations and efficacy issues. Additionally, the influence of community attitudes toward integration of handicapped individuals into community settings is discussed. Directions for the future are based on recommendations in the literature and a conceptual framework for examining factors which influence service delivery. The framework is drawn from the sociological literature and addresses variables of human behavior at three levels (a) the micro-analytic level, (b) the meso-analytic level, and (c) the macro-analytic level. The discussion provides direction for new research designs which address factors at one or more levels using single subject as well as group designs. Recommendations are included for behavioral research addressing the system as a whole and the development of a technology for positive change.

The passage and implementation of P.L. 94-142, The Education of All Handicapped Act of 1975, marked the advent of a new era with regard to the treatment of exceptional children and youth. Dur-

---

Patt Kearly is affiliated with the Education Transition Center, 650 University Avenue, #200, Sacramento, CA 95825.

3

ing the 1970s and early 1980s, dramatic shifts in philosophical approach resulted in marked changes in both political policies and social practices affecting the handicapped. This chapter will present a summary of historical perspectives which have influenced past practice and the guiding principles which influence present service delivery. The concept of "normalization" as an underlying principle will be reviewed and issues related to community integration will be discussed. Finally, recommendations for future directions at the individual level, the organizational level and the community level will be presented.

HISTORICAL PERSPECTIVES REGARDING THE HANDICAPPED

The philosophical beliefs which characterize society at a given point in time have had a profound effect on treatment of special populations. Hewett and Forness (1974) have suggested that four factors have served as major influences on societal views of deviancy (a) the influence of superstition, (b) the influence of economic and social forces related to survival, (c) the influence of societal attitudes regarding service and human rights, and (d) the influence of science and technology.

The influence of changing societal attitudes on human services has been discussed at length by Rhodes (1975). The shifting theoretical approaches to child variance have suggested a movement away from narrow definitions of "normality," to societal integration of wider degrees of difference into the range of acceptable adaptive behavior. Rhodes predicted that efforts to delabel and increase client participation in decision-making were probable outcomes if the helping process were viewed as social ritual leading to policies rather than mutual problem-solving leading to solutions.

In a similar vein, Burello and Sage (1979) have emphasized the social systems perspective in their discussion of leadership and change in special education. These authors have suggested that although the treatment of handicapped individuals is influenced by factors internal to the educational system, the most potent forces for change are rooted in factors external to the boundaries of the educational system. From within a social systems framework (Getzels &

Guba, 1957; Getzels, Lipham, & Campbell, 1968), the general social climate as manifested by litigation and legislation is viewed as a primary factor in the change process. Burello and Sage have suggested that over time, changes in the general social climate have led to tolerance for a wider degree of variation in human behavior as evidenced in a variety of social contexts.

> The normalization ideology, which provides the philosophic base for the deinstitutionalization and mainstreaming practices in public schools, is the specific manifestation of this force in the context of services for the handicapped. (Burello & Sage, 1979, p. 34)

The treatment of the handicapped has been influenced over time by changing societal attitudes and other economic, cultural, and political factors. A number of writers in the field have attempted to identify specific eras in treatment philosophy (Kauffman & Payne, 1975; Kolstoe & Frey, 1965). The following section outlines an expanded historical perspective which includes seven distinct eras of treatment: (a) the era of extermination, (b) the era of ridicule, (c) the era of asylum, (d) the era of hope for education, (e) the era of disillusionment, (f) the era of integration, and (g) the era of technology.

The Era of Extermination

In the evolutionary notion of historical development, primitive societies were dependent upon the fitness of their members to contribute to community survival. Individuals who were unable to contribute were not only viewed as less valuable, but were viewed as a burden and a potential risk to the overall survival of the group. Handicapped children were killed at birth as a matter of common practice. In ancient Greece defective children were banished to the outskirts of the city and left to die. The philosophy underlying the practice of extermination at birth of deformed children has been traditionally based on a notions of "incurability" and "inability to contribute to the common good."

The Era of Ridicule

The historical development of the agrarian caste system resulted in a decrease in the emphasis on survival as the primary mode of operation. Basic safety requirements of noblemen and serfs were more stable as communities developed around the manors of ruling class. Handicapped individuals were tolerated as the lowest class in the society, one step above extermination, but not above ridicule. The roles of the "town fool" and the "court jester" were commonly filled by mentally or physically handicapped people (Dunn, 1973). The philosophy underlying the practice of ridicule has been traditionally based on a notion of "class" where deviancy from the norm provides a basis for discrimination and justification for denial of basic human rights.

The Era of Asylum

Society's view of the handicapped underwent a gradual shift during the Middle Ages. The primary influence for this changing philosophy was provided by the Catholic Church. The emergence of a belief in moral treatment of the handicapped as "children of God" resulted in the development of asylums run by nuns or monks affiliated with various religious orders. Handicapped people were provided with shelter and minimal custodial care under the aegis of the church. The philosophy underlying the practice of asylum has traditionally been based on the notion of "separatism" where provision of care was viewed as most properly provided in a setting separate from the mainstream of society.

The Era of Hope for Education

The concept of education for handicapped individuals was vastly influenced by Itard (1962), who in 1799 documented an attempt to educate a feral child. The 11- to 12-year-old wild boy (Victor) was found wandering in the woods of France with no ability to speak or respond to verbal instruction. Although Itard's attempts to normalize Victor were less than totally successful, the case study provided the impetus for educational efforts with various categories of handicapped individuals. Schools for the deaf and the blind were started initially in Europe and were later used as models for American development in the late 1800s and early 1900s. The era of hope for education was based on a philosophy that a "cure" was possible and that through training, handicapped individuals could become "contributing members of society."

The Era of Disillusionment

During the early 1900s hopes continued to be high that educational treatment could cure the problems created by handicapping conditions. When these efforts were met with only minimal success, treatment of the handicapped began to reflect the faltering of philosophy. Where once institutions were viewed as "islands of hope" these structures became "islands of desolation." Perhaps the most vivid portrayal of this situation was depicted in a publication by Blatt and Kaplan (1966) entitled *Christmas in Purgatory: A Photographic Essay on Mental Retardation*. The realities of institutional practice were presented in black and white and contrasted against the Christmas holiday season on glossy pages for all to see. The philosophy of education was overshadowed by disillusionment and institutionalization with less than adequate care becoming common practice.

The Era of Integration

It was during the mid 1900s that societal practices regarding the handicapped were contested in the courts. Parents of retarded individuals had joined forces in 1950 to form a national association (presently known as the National Association for Retarded Citizens) concerned with promoting services and rights for the handicapped. The standard of "separate but equal" as a racial issue was brought to the Supreme Court in Brown vs. the Board of Education in 1954. The principle from this case was later extended via litigation to justify the right to free appropriate education for the handicapped. Included within the litigation was the notion of the least restrictive environment as a means for providing opportunity for "normal" interaction between the handicapped and their nonhandicapped peers.

The social climate of the times was further influenced by political forces as manifested by the efforts of the Kennedy family. The President's Committee on Mental Retardation was established in 1966 to promote planning and implementation of community centered programs for the mentally retarded. The influence of political, legal, and social forces eventually led to major legislation in 1975 to mandate education of all handicapped children.

The philosophy underlying the era of integration was based on the principle of normalization (Nirje, 1969; Wolfensberger, 1972). The principle includes the assumption that availability of culturally normative patterns and conditions of everyday living to handicapped individuals will lead to more culturally normative behavior. Manifestations of this changing philosophy can be noted in the de-institutionalization movement of the early 1970s. Mainstreaming, the practice of integrating handicapped students into physical settings with their nonhandicapped peers for educational purposes, also had its origins in this time period.

The Era of Technology

The basic principles of behaviorism which serve as the foundation for the era of technology are most closely associated with the work of Skinner (1938). His experiments with operant conditioning were carried out using laboratory animals as subjects. Later researchers (Ayllon, 1963; Ayllon & Azrin, 1964; Barrett & Lindsey, 1962; Bijou, 1963, 1966; Giradeau & Spradlin, 1964; Lindsey, 1956, 1960; Zeaman, House, & Orlando, 1958) employed behavioristic principles in their research on human behavior. The behavioristic model assumes that maladaptive behaviors are learned and maintained in the same ways as are more adaptive behaviors. The model differs from the medical and developmental models in that it is not concerned with internal events or original causes, but rather focuses on antecedent and consequent stimuli in the present environment.

It was not until the late 1960s and early 1970s that applied behavior analysis techniques began to receive serious attention in the psychological literature. The philosophical differences between the behavioristic/behavioral model and the more common models led to strong controversy in the field. The implications for direct systematic action and the emphasis on observable effect led to rapid adoption of the behavioral model by many service providers.

The influence of applied behavior analysis has forced those involved in the field to closely examine the assumptions and the long-term effects of current practices. Legal and ethical issues regarding the rights of the handicapped have been brought to the forefront. The uses and misuses of punishment in changing behavior have fueled the fires of those opposed to the use of behavioral technology. Assumptions around the normalization principle have been questioned especially with regard to the use of "ordinary means" to establish normative behavior in the mentally regarded.

The philosophy underlying the era of technology is based on the assumption that providing opportunity for interaction with nonhandicapped peers is necessary, but not sufficient, for establishing and maintaining normative behavior for many handicapped individuals. The philosophy has forced service providers to examine the issue of transfer as an essential element in community integration. Focus has shifted to development of long-term strategies for maintenance of social skills and adaptive behaviors in the natural environment.

The changing historical perspectives which have affected services for the handicapped provide a backdrop for examination of the theoretical foundations which undergird present practice. The normalization principle has been a major influence in the field and a discussion of its origins and implications has bearing on community integration for the handicapped.

NORMALIZATION:
THE ROOTS OF PRESENT PRACTICE

Origins and Assumptions

The concept of normalization found its way into American philosophy through the influence provided by the Scandinavian countries. A delegation of representatives from the United States visited several European countries in the early 1960s and were very favorably impressed with the Scandinavian attitudes and services for the handicapped. The original concept was rooted in Danish legislation concerned with services for the mentally retarded. The normalization principle and its implications for service were later summarized by Nirje (1969) under the sponsorship of the President's Committee on Mental Retardation. Nirje's definition focused on opportunity for exposure to "patterns and conditions of everyday life which are as close as possible to the norms and patterns of the mainstream of society" (Nirje, 1969, p. 181). Inherent within this definition is the assumption that the norms and patterns of mainstream society are patterns which handicapped individuals should pursue. Further, there is an assumption that exposure to "normality" will lead to changes in behavior for the mentally retarded.

Presently, one of the most widely quoted definitions of the concept of normalization is that provided by Wolfensberger (1972): "Utilization of means which are as culturally normative as possible, in order to establish and/or maintain personal behaviors and characteristics which are as culturally normative as possible" (Wolfensberger, 1972, p. 28). This definition focuses on two dimensions; the means and the ends. It emphasizes the goal of establishing and maintaining normative behavior, but at the same time suggests that the means should be limited to practices common to the cultural context. Inherent within this definition is the implication that the least restrictive environments for establishing normative behavior are the conditions common to the cultural context. Secondly, the definition assumes that "normal" methods can be effective in establishing normative behavior.

A number of writers have logically argued that for many handicapped individuals utilization of normative means is not the most effective way to achieve the goal of normative behavior (Aanes & Haagenson, 1978; Roos, 1972; Miller, 1974; Throne, 1979). The critics of Wolfensberger argue that normal means are not adequate for helping the retarded to achieve higher degrees of functioning and that extraordinary methods must be employed to achieve more normal behavior in retarded individuals (Throne, 1975). In many cases, deinstitutionalization and mainstreaming practices have been based on the assumption that mere exposure to nonhandicapped peers (physical integration) will result in positive behavioral change, thus reducing the degree of social retardation. However, other researchers (Marchetti & Matson, 1981; Matson, 1980; Neef, Iwata, & Page, 1978; Rusch, Connis, & Sowers, 1979; Rusch &

Kazdin, 1981; VandePol et al., 1981; Vogelsburg & Rusch, 1979) have provided convincing evidence that utilization of specialized techniques is essential for establishing behavioral change and promoting response maintenance of skills necessary for community survival (social integration) with mentally retarded individuals.

Other writers (Hendrix, 1981; Mesibov, 1976; Rhoades & Browning, 1977) have argued that assumptions about normalization and the least restrictive environment are based on value systems of the nonhandicapped society. It has been contended that the normalization principle has been used as the rationale for "dumping" retarded individuals into environments where they are physically integrated with nonhandicapped individuals, but emotionally isolated from contact with persons exhibiting similar disabilities. It has been suggested that current practices have been geared toward the needs of agencies, not clients, and normalization has been used as a banner to give respectability to less than adequate service.

Implications for Community Integration

Wolfensberger (1980) has suggested that criticisms levied at the normalization principle are based on misunderstanding. He contends that the goal of normalization is to provide culturally valued treatment which he terms as "social role valorization." He suggests that extraordinary measures may be necessary to establish normative behavior. He cautions that reason should be employed to assure that the potential for "damage" through utilization of nonnormative measures does not outweigh the potential for positive change. Further, he suggests that true integration should include development of intimate social relationships with nonhandicapped individuals.

In spite of the criticisms which surround the normalization notion, the principle has served as the primary basis for service provision to the handicapped. Wolfensberger has listed five implications for residential services based on the normalization principle. He has suggested that group residential facilities should: (a) be integrated with easy accessibility to the community; (b) be small; (c) be specialized to serve individuals with similar degrees of need for supervision; (d) serve strictly as homes and not serve dually as work sites; and (e) provide a continuum of services based on need. The implications from Wolfensberger's work are thus, closely related to the practice of deinstitutionalization.

Similarly related to the principle of normalization is the practice of mainstreaming in the educational setting. The effect of the civil rights movement in the late 1950s and early 1960s led to examination of the practices related to the education of the handicapped. The justifiability of separate education for the handicapped came under strict fire (Dunn, 1968; Goldstein, Moss, & Jordon, 1965; MacMillan, Jones, & Aloia, 1974; Mercer, 1973). In the early 1970s equal educational opportunity within the normal societal structure became a major legal issue.

ISSUES FOR CONSIDERATION

Legal and Ethical Issues

The civil rights movement beginning with Brown vs. Board of Education resulted in reexamination of the rights of minorities. The litigation stemming from this movement included court cases regarding mentally retarded individuals. In 1972, Wyatt vs. Stickney became a landmark case dealing with the "right to treatment" and minimum standards of care for institutionalized mentally retarded individuals. The ruling by Judge Johnson, not only addressed deficiencies in the quantity and quality of service delivery at Partlow State School and Hospital, but also included statements of philosophy related to the normalization principle.

Another issue included within the caselaw dealing with the mentally retarded has involved the "right to protection from harm." In 1975, the case of The New York Association for Retarded Children vs. Carey included requirements for the establishment of community facilities to accommodate a majority of the residents of the Willowbrook Developmental Center. The consent decree resulting from the case included reference to the concept of restrictiveness related to the environmental setting.

As a result of precedents set by a number of caselaw decisions, the philosophy of the normalization principle has been embedded in current legislation regarding mentally handicapped individuals. Legislation such as The Developmental Disabilities Act (P.L. 94-103) and The Education for All Handicapped Act (P.L. 94-142) incorporate the normalization principle through requirements for service in the least restrictive environment.

While most professionals do not disagree with inclusion of the goals of normalization into legislative language, the issue of means as to how the goals should be achieved has been an extremely controversial one. Nonbehaviorists have contended that only through the use of culturally normative means can habilitation be achieved. Behaviorists have countered that there is no evidence to support the notion that "only through culturally normative means" can normal behavior be achieved. It has been argued instead that normal methods have obviously been ineffective in establishing behavior which conforms to the norms and patterns of everyday life. It has been further argued that in some cases, the withholding of extraordinary means to eliminate maladaptive behavior (i.e., self-abuse) could be interpreted as a violation of the right to protection from harm.

Unfortunately, the issue of means has been incorporated into legislative langauge further complicating requirements for service delivery. This trend for legislative interpretation of what constitutes sound practice has been staunchly criticized by McCarver and Cavalier (1983). Siding with the position articulated by Judge Johnson in the continuing Wyatt litigation (Wyatt vs. Ireland, 1979), McCarver and Cavalier hold that while it is the province of the court to determine constitutional rights for the mentally retarded, determination of means for actualization should be left in the hands of *social scientists*, not judges.

The legal and ethical issues related to treatment of retarded individuals have focused on individual rights, the goals of treatment, and values concerning the means of treatment. The basic issue in almost all cases has been a question of power and control. The use of treatment techniques designed to predict and control the behavior of retarded individuals has raised serious ethical questions in the field (Braun, 1975; Roos, 1974).

By the mid-1970s, increased attention by the public to legal and ethical issues surrounding the use of behavior modification resulted in the development of standards and guidelines for the use of behavioral techniques with the retarded by a number of organizations. In 1975 the American Association on Mental Deficiency (AAMD) published a policy statement discussing the issues of informed consent, program review, and monitoring of individual habilitation plans (AAMD, 1975). Around the same time, the National Association for Retarded Citizens (NARC) developed and adopted a set of guidelines for the use of behavior modification procedures in residential settings (NARC, 1975). Included with this document were specific recommendations for procedural operation, program review, and steps for obtaining informed consent. In a somewhat less specific vein, ethical issues in using behavior modification techniques were addressed in guidelines published in 1977 by the American Association for Advancement of Behavior Therapy (AABT, 1977). Shortly thereafter, another set of standards was published by the Accreditation Council for Services for Mentally Retarded and Other Developmentally Disabled Persons (1978).

Based on a review of various state guidelines, Morris and Brown (1983) proposed a three level system for use of behavior modification techniques with mentally retarded persons. The proposed system includes three levels and assumes that the degree of intrusiveness associated with a Level I procedure (e.g., implementation of a token economy system) is less than the level of intrusiveness associated with a procedure at Level II (e.g., response cost) or Level III (e.g., overcorrection). The authors recommend that a hierarchical implementation process be employed, and that service providers should obtain informed consent and both internal and external reviews of treatment plans on an ongoing basis.

Presently, most agencies operate under a specific set of guidelines which define the level of intrusiveness or restrictiveness of various intervention techniques. Most systems include limitations and requirements for both internal and external review of behavioral procedures on an individual basis. The restrictions placed on use of behavioral procedures have been aimed at preventing misuse of power with retarded individuals. The issue of effectiveness of treatment (when less intrusive procedures are employed prior to the use of more restrictive interventions) has been "noticeably avoided."

Efficacy Issues

One of the major concerns voiced by proponents of behavioral programming has been that comparable procedures of review have not been implemented for less controversial treatment strategies (Morris & Brown, 1983). The behaviorists argue that the efficacy of many of the nonbehavioral strategies is highly questionable and that limitations placed on the use of interventions with demonstrated effectiveness will retard progress in the development of behavioral technology in community settings.

The research on empirical benefits derived from community-based placement has been mixed. Comparisons are complicated by a lack of agreement on what constitutes benefit and the criteria for its evaluation (Lakin, Bruininks, & Sigford, 1981). In some cases, community placement may include the notion of competitive employment. In other cases benefit may be simply defined as maintenance within a community residential facility. The wide diversity among community facilities on variables such as size, client characteristics, and other organizational structures make comparisons of both quantity and quality extremely difficult (Baker, Seltzer & Seltzer, 1977; Balla, 1976; Baroff, 1980; Crawford, Aiello, & Thompson, 1979; George & Baumeister, 1981).

In spite of these methodological problems, research findings strongly support the effectiveness of a behavioral technology for modifying maladaptive behaviors and establishing repertoires of new behaviors (Cuvo & Davis, 1983). Studies in community settings have suggested that significant changes in adaptive behavior are related to environmental factors and do not occur without specialized programming (Eyman, Silverstein, McLain, & Miller, 1977; Aninger & Bilinsky, 1977).

Community Attitudes

Community attitudes have also been recognized as a highly potent factor in community placement for handicapped individuals. Basically, research in this area has been of two types: (a) research on attitudes for hypothetical situations; and (b) research on attitudes where group homes have been established. The research on expressed attitudes toward hypothetical community placement of mentally retarded persons has been very inconsistent (Kastner, Repucci, & Pezzoli, 1979; Margolis & Charitonidis, 1981; President's Committee on Mental Retardation, 1975; Smith, 1981; Trippi, Michael, Colao, & Alverez, 1978; Willms, 1978). The validity of this body of research has been questioned in terms of its potential for bias and its relationship to actual behavior.

Other researchers have assessed the perceptions of residents, staff, and nonhandicapped community members where group homes have actually been established. Okolo and Guskin (1984) have noted that in three large scale studies (Baker, Seltzer, & Seltzer, 1977; Gollay, Freedman, Wyngaarden, & Kurtz, 1978; O'Connor, 1976), representative sampling procedures were employed with various individuals and in two cases (Baker et al., 1977; O'Connor, 1976) the organization was used as the unit of analysis. Findings from these studies were consistent in showing that community attitudes constitute a significant problem in community placement.

Research has also suggested that community attitudes may strongly influence the actual degree of social integration experienced by handicapped individuals residing in community placements (Segal & Aviram, 1978) or the geographic location of the facility (Chandler & Ross, 1976; Lauber & Bangs, 1974). Data from a number of studies have suggested that "isolation in the mainstream" is a pattern of living for many handicapped individuals and that this pattern does not improve with time (Birenbaum & Re, 1979; Schalock, Harper, & Carver, 1981).

Many variables have been examined as possible *barriers* to community placement. Some of these variables have included (a) community objections to the racial and sexual composition of the facility, (b) fears about the potential for sexual deviance in the residents, (c) fears about the potential for increased crime in the area, and (d) fears about the potential for a drop in neighborhood property values (Berdiansky & Parker, 1977; Segal & Aviram, 1978).

Negative attitudes appear to persist in spite of research which refutes the actualization of fears surrounding the establishment of a community facility. The research does not support the notion that placement of retarded clients in community settings results in increased crime or other norm-violating behavior (Mamula & Newman, 1973; Sitkei, 1980). Similarly, community attitudes related to property devaluation with the advent of a community facility appear to be unfounded (Dear, 1977; Weiner, Anderson, & Nietupski, 1982).

Parental opposition to deinstitutionalization for handicapped individuals has also been researched and documented in legal action as a barrier to community placement (Halderman vs. Pennhurst, 1977; Hill & Wehman, 1980; Meyer, 1980; Scheerenberger, 1978). Parental attitudes have been related to concerns about quality of care and lack of adequate community services (Meyer, 1980).

Okolo and Guskin (1984) have suggested that parental opposition is understandable when one considers the historical counsel received by many of the families of handicapped children and it may be justifiable in areas where negative community attitudes are strong. Okolo and Guskin have noted that most research on the topic of community placement has been based on assumptions that quality of life for handicapped individuals will be more satisfying in community settings and that greater exposure to handicapped individuals will decrease resistance to community placement. They suggest that future research should include longitudinal case studies which employ qualitative data analysis and multiple data sources.

The legal-ethical, attitudinal, and efficacy issues related to community placement for the mentally handicapped provide a stage from which future directions for programming and research can be viewed. Implications are related to individual, organizational, and community levels of analysis.

DIRECTIONS

The current literature dealing with training for handicapped individuals offers a number of suggestions for future research on community placement for the handicapped. The following section provides a brief summary of the primary recommendations provided in two recent reviews, and describes a conceptual framework from which research implications for the future can be drawn.

Recommendations in the Literature

The issues which have been associated with the transition from highly restrictive settings to alternative living arrangements in the community, have been related to a number of variables affecting the success of community placement for handicapped individuals. Much of the research with both children and older handicapped individuals has focused on development of functional skills related to community integration. Specific areas of concentration have included skills in self-care, mobility, interpersonal communication, independent living, and structuring of leisure time activities. More recently, researchers have given attention to the concept of generalization of skills into the community setting. Two important reviews in the literature have provided direction for future research efforts.

Cuvo and Davis (1983) published an extensive review of the empirical research on the use of behavioral techniques to develop community living skills with handicapped individuals. Specific skills addressed in the studies included (a) self-care skills, (b) safety skills, (c) monetary skills, (d) mobility skills, and (e) telephone skills. After reviewing more than 40 studies, these authors highly recommended that future research address clients' environments of ultimate functioning:

> It is essential that researchers demonstrate that clients actually can perform the skill trained in the community setting under naturally occurring conditions. If skills are taught using artificial or simulated settings and materials, transfer of stimulus control procedures to natural environmental conditions are [will be] essential elements in a program. (Cuvo & Davis, 1983, p. 166)

The authors have offered additional recommendations concerning assessment through direct observation of skills needed in the natural environment. It was suggested that the social validity of skills selected for training be established by input from service providers and community members. Noting the terminology of previous writers (Brown, Nietupski, & Hamre-Nietupski, 1976; Vincent, Salisburg, Walter, Brown, Grunewald, & Powers, 1980), it was recommended that the criterion for success should reflect the level required in the environment into which the handicapped individual will ultimately be placed. Additionally, replicability issues related to staffing ratios and prompting transfer of stimulus control were discussed. The use of treatment withdrawal designs proposed by Rusch and Kazdin (1981) were suggested to promote efficient behavioral maintenance.

A second review provided by Jacobson and Schwartz (1983) focused on the effects of community residential living for developmentally disabled individuals. The authors discussed research on various characteristics of community residences as well as characteristics of the clients served. Other factors such as staff job satisfaction, quality of care, and program costs were also addressed. Jacobson and Schwartz (1983) concluded that: (a) mentally retarded individuals can benefit from placement in community residential facilities if appropriate interventional strategies are employed; (b) the restrictiveness of the setting is related to the degree of skill attainment; and (c) characteristics of the community residence are strongly associated with success or failure of the placement. Additionally, the authors have provided a model system for evaluating community residences and have offered suggestions for appropriate measures in group home research.

A Conceptual Framework

The conceptual framework offered as a perspective for future research on community placement for the handicapped is derived from the sociological literature and employs the terminology of Hage (1980). Three distinct levels of analysis are envisioned as important in the assessment of human behavior. The three levels are identified as (a) the micro-analytic level, (b) the meso-analytic level, and (c) the macro-analytic level.

At the micro-analytic level, individuals serve as the unit of analysis and characteristics associated with a number of children or a given child could be assessed. Functional living skills for a given child are examples of behavior at this level. At the meso-analytic level, organizations or subgroups of organizations serve as the unit of analysis and characteristics associated with a number of community residences, a given type of residential home, or a given community residence could be assessed. Size of the residence(s), level of centralization, staff to client interaction ratios, or other types of measures associated with the organizational unit are examples of variables at this level. At the macro-analytic level, environments or subgroups of environments serve as the unit of analysis. Characteristics associated with a number of communities or neighborhoods or a given community or neighborhood could be assessed. Community reactions to plans for establishment of a group home or tolerance levels to deviant behavior in a given neighborhood could be variables at the environmental level. A visual depiction of this multi-level model is presented in Figure 1.

This multilevel model is based on the assumption that minimally acceptable levels of adaptive behavior are necessary but not sufficient to insure successful community integration for a given indi-

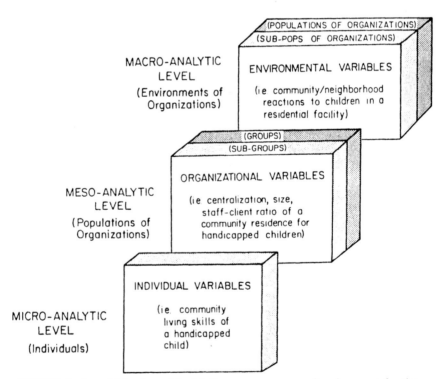

FIGURE 1. A multi-level model of influences on community placement for the handicapped.

vidual. The model suggests that factors at the organizational and community levels of analysis also exert influence on individuals and manipulation of variables at these levels may be necessary to bring about successful generalization of skills and long-term community integration. It is assumed that reciprocity of influence exists both between and within levels. It is not assumed however, that the multiple factors at each level exert equal influence on behavior. Finally, it is assumed that characteristics associated with a community facility at the organizational level of analysis exert a significant influence on the behavior of individual residents (Bjaanes, Butler, & Kelly, 1981; Kanter, 1977; Schinke & Wong, 1977).

The underlying theoretical premises of the model are based on sociological principles derived from organizational research in a variety of settings. The model is based on the premise that a community residence is an open system which is receptive to influences from the community in which it exists and in turn exerts influence on that community (Aiken & Hage, 1967). A second premise assumes that behavior within organizational boundaries is rational (Scott, 1981). Thirdly, it is presumed that residential facilities are loosely-coupled systems (Weick, 1976) characterized by differential capacities to process information from the environment at various locations within the organization.

The conceptual framework provides a perspective for viewing influences at different levels within the total system. Within the behavioral research to date, most studies have focused on variables at the individual level to the exclusion of variables at the organizational or community levels of analysis. Some writers (Brown, Branston, Hamre-Nietupski, Pumpian, Certo, & Grunewald, 1979; Brown, Branston-McClean, Baumgart, Vincent, Falvey, & Schroeder, 1979) have discussed the importance of assessing environmental characteristics and establishing a functional curriculum for given handicapped individuals based on the skills necessary for maintenance in the anticipated placement. The emphasis of the Brown model is on programming for individual transitions to less restrictive settings, but attention is not aimed at manipulation of organizational or environmental variables.

The tendency to ignore community and organizational factors in behavioral research has been noted by a growing number of writers in the field (Butler & Bjaanes, 1977; Jacobson & Schwartz, 1983;

Jones, Risley & Favell, 1983; Novak & Berkeley, 1984; O'Donnell, 1977; Willms, 1978). Marchetti and Matson (1981) have suggested that a major problem in behavioral research has been an emphasis on treatment techniques to enhance individual performance to the exclusion of attention on improvement on service delivery systems. Additionally, the authors note a lack of attention to staff training and community attitudes.

This framework suggests conceptualization of future research analyzing factors at one or more levels using single subject as well as group designs. Assessment and research considerations at each of the three levels are complicated due to a variety of factors. Future research must be carefully designed to control for methodological problems related to both reliability and validity.

Directions at the Individual Level

The research on training community adjustment skills at the individual level of analysis has included a wide range of behaviors including self-care skills, daily living skills, leisure skills, communication, and related social skills. It has been noted, however, that much of the research has been methodologically weak (Marchetti & Matson, 1981) with inadequate descriptions to allow for replication studies. Additionally, more attention needs to be focused on training for response generalization and maintenance in the natural environment over time. The increasing interest in sequential withdrawal designs (Kazdin, 1982; Rusch & Kazdin, 1981) for assessment of response maintenance is an encouraging sign in the literature.

Directions at the Organizational Level

Much of the early research on organizational factors has been published in the sociological literature and has been descriptive and/or correlational in nature. A number of problems have been noted in this research and have resulted in mixed findings.

Most of this research on organizational characteristics has employed group designs and only a portion (Blau & Schoenherr, 1971; Pugh, Hickson, Hinings, & Turner, 1969) of this research has relied on objective measures of organizational variables. In contrast, some researchers have relied on subjective measures as more valid indicators of organizational characteristics (Aiken & Hage, 1968).

Pennings (1973), however, found low intercorrelations between objective and subjective measures of organizational structure and suggested that different dimensions of organizations may be relevant to research on structure.

Another problem in the past research on organizations has been that operational definitions of organizational characteristics and levels of analysis across studies have been inconsistent. For example, the variable of size has been treated by some investigators as a dependent variable indicative of demand at the environmental level (Blau & Schoenherr, 1971; Pugh et al., 1969), while others have treated size as an independent variable (Aldrich, 1972; Kearly, 1984) at the organizational level of analysis. Size has also been measured using different indicators (number of beds, number of clients, net assets) with the most common being number of participants (Kimberly, 1976).

Researchers directly interested in aspects of community placement have focused on variables such as employee job satisfaction, staff interaction patterns, participation in decision-making and quality of care (Holland, 1973; Landesman-Dwyer, Sackett, & Kleinman, 1980; MacEachron & Driscoll, 1981; Pratt, Luszcz, & Brown, 1980). Although much of the research in these areas has been methodologically weak, the findings consistently support a relationship between organizational variables and dependent variables related to quality of care.

As we become more technologically skilled in modifying human behavior, it is imperative that we begin to address behavioral change at the organizational level. Studies at this level might identify one organization as the single subject for analysis where manipulation of a selected independent variable is planned. In the long run we will need to identify those variables which influence overall service delivery and address qualitative issues at the "heart" of our science (Wolf, 1978).

Implications at the Environmental Level

Research at the environmental level related to community integration for the mentally retarded has been limited. As noted in the recent literature (Nirhira, Mink, & Meyers, 1984) only four standardized scales for environmental assessment have been commonly used in the research. These are Wolfensberger and Glenn's (1975) Program Analysis of Service Systems (PASS); the Moo's Scales (1975); the Characteristics of Treatment Environment Scale (Jackson, 1969); and the Residential Management Scale (King, Raynes, & Tizard, 1971). For a description of research conducted with standardized instruments the reader is referred to Novak and Berkeley (1984).

Most of the studies which have been conducted at the environmental level have employed group designs and have focused on concepts such as normalization, client care practices, family structures, and quality of care. Future research efforts should attempt to operationally define variables at the environmental level which exert influence on community attitudes and factors which affect response maintenance for handicapped individuals in the natural setting.

Additionally, single-case analysis at the environmental level could be conducted with characteristics of a given group home serving as the dependent variables. This type of research would necessarily be based on assumptions about group home characteristics and their subsequent influence on client behavior. A study at this level could involve the development of a community media training package designed to prepare a community for reception of a group home in a given neighborhood. The study might test the community reception training package across three neighborhoods using a multiple baseline to establish the efficacy of the package as a facilitator of transition to normal environments for handicapped individuals. Assumptions about client behaviors could be tested as a follow-up (Experiment 2) to the initial study.

CONCLUSIONS AND RECOMMENDATIONS

There are many reasons why research at the organizational and environmental levels has not been extensive. First, research at the individual level of analysis is the most obvious and the most easily manipulated for the purposes of research. Secondly, the identification of key variables at the organizational and environmental levels is problematic when one considers the complexity involved in assessing multiple variables at multiple levels. Thirdly, the research to date has employed both objective and subjective measures which has made analysis of findings difficult. Similarly, concepts have been operationalized using different definitions. Sometimes concepts have been assigned as dependent variables and at other times the same concepts have been treated as independent variables. Finally, factors at the organizational and environmental levels are not easily alterable and are thus, most commonly assessed using *ex post facto* analyses such as correlational studies or factor analysis. Missing from the research are single-case studies at the organizational and/or environmental levels of analysis.

The shifting philosophical perspectives which have shaped policy and practice toward handicapped people in our society have placed us in an era of technology. We have developed knowledge and skills for the modification of behavior based on principles of learning. However,

> while there are established techniques to change the behavior of the individual, there exists no thorough and systematic understanding of how to activate, move, and alter the larger levels constructing the system which surrounds the individual. (Novak & Berkeley, 1984)

The literature has offered us models for evaluation (Jacobson & Schwartz, 1983) and strategies for exploration (Thompson & Wray, 1985). The challenge for the future is to research those factors which significantly influence the system as a whole and develop a technology for positive change.

REFERENCES

Aanes, D., & Haagenson, L. (1978). Normalization: Attention to a conceptual disaster. *Mental Retardation, 16*, 55-56.

Accreditation Council for Services for Mentally Retarded and other Developmentally Disabled Persons (1978). *Standards for services for developmentally disabled individuals.* Chicago: Joint Commission on Accreditation of Hospitals.

Aiken, M., & Hage, J. (1967). Organizational alienation: A comparative analysis. *American Sociological Review, 31*, 497-507.

Aiken, M., & Hage, J. (1968). Organizational Interdependence and intra-organizational structure. *American Sociological Review, 33*, 912-931.

Aldrich, H. E. (1972). Technology and organizational structure: A reexamination of the findings of the Aston group. *Administrative Science Quarterly, 17*, 26-43.

American Association for Advancement of Behavior Therapy (1977). Ethical issues for human services. *Behavior Therapy, 8*, v-vi.

American Association on Mental Deficiency (1975). Human rights review and protection boards. *Mental Retardation, 13*, vi-viii.

Aninger, M., & Bilinsky, K. (1977). Levels of independent functioning of retarded adults in apartments. *Mental Retardation, 15*, 12-16.

Ayllon, T. (1963). Intensive treatment of psychotic behavior by stimulus satiation and food reinforcement. *Behavior Research and Therapy, 1*, 53-61.

Ayllon, T., & Azrin, N. H. (1964). Reinforcement and instructions with mental patients. *Journal of the Experimental Analysis of Behavior, 7*, 327-331.

Baker, B. L., & Seltzer, G. B., & Seltzer, M. M. (1977). *As close as possible: A study of community residences for retarded adults*. Boston: Little, Brown.

Balla, D. (1976). Relationship of institution size to quality of care: A review of the literature. *American Journal of Mental Deficiency, 81*, 117-124.

Baroff, G. (1980). On "size" and the quality of residential care: A second look. *Mental Retardation, 18*, 113-118.

Barrett, B., & Lindsey, O. R. (1962). Deficits in acquisition of operant discrimination and differentiation shown by institutionalized retarded children. *American Journal of Mental Deficiency, 67*, 424-426.

Berdiansky, H. A., & Parker, R. (1977). Establishing a group home for the adult mentally retarded in North Carolina. *Mental Retardation, 15*, 8-11.

Bijou, S. W. (1963). Theory and research in mental (developmental) retardation. *The Psychological Record, 13*, 95-110.

Bijou, S. W. (1966). A functional analysis of retarded development. In N. R. Ellis (Ed.), *International review of research on mental retardation* (Vol. 1). New York: Academic Press.

Birenbaum, A., & Re, M. A. *Resetting retarded adults in a managed community*. New York: Praeger.

Bjaanes, A. T., Butler, D. W., & Kelly, B. R. (1981). Placement type and client functional level as factors in provision of services aimed at increasing adjustment. In R. H. Bruininks, C. E. Myers, B. B. Sigford, & K. C. Lakin (Eds.), *Deinstitutionalization and community adjustment of mentally retarded people*. Washington, DC: American Association on Mental Deficiency.

Blatt, B. S., & Kaplan, F. (1966). *Christmas in purgatory: A photographic essay on mental retardation*. Boston: Allyn & Bacon.

Blau, P. M., & Schoenherr, R. A. (1971). *The structure of organizations*. New York: Basic Books.

Braun, S. H. (1975). Ethical issues in behavior modification. *Behavior Therapy, 6*, 51-62.

Brown, L., Branston-McClean, M. B., Baumgart, D., Vincent, L., Falvey, M., & Schroeder, J. (1979). Using the characteristics of current and subsequent least restrictive environments as factors in the development of curricular content for severely handicapped students. *AAESPH Review, 4*, 407-424.

Brown, L., Branston, M. B., Hamre-Nietupski, S., Pumpian, I., Certo, N., & Gruenewald, L. (1979). A strategy for developing chronological-age-appropriate and functional curricular content for severely handicapped adolescents and young adults. *The Journal of Special Education, 13,* 81-90.

Brown, L., Nietupski, J., & Hamre-Nietupski, S. (1976). The criterion of ultimate functioning and public school services for the severely handicapped student. In A. Thomas (Ed.), *Hey don't forget about me: Education's investment in the severely, profoundly and multiply handicapped.* Reston, VA: Council for Exceptional Children.

Brown vs. Board of Education, 347, U.S., 483, (1954).

Burello, L. C., & Sage, D. D. (1979). *Leadership and change in special education.* Englewood Cliffs, NJ: Prentice-Hall.

Butler, E. W., & Bjaanes, A. T. (1977). A typology of community care facilities and differential normalization outcomes. In P. Mittler (Ed.), *Research to practice in mental retardation: Care and intervention.* Baltimore, MD: University Park Press.

Chandler, J., & Ross, S. (1976). Zoning restrictions and the right to live in the community. In M. Kindred, J. Cohen, D. Penrod, & T. Shaffer (Eds.), *The mentally retarded citizen and the law.* New York: Free Press.

Crawford, J. L., Aiello, J. R., & Thompson, D.E. (1979). Deinstitutionalization and community placement: Clinical and environmental factors. *Mental Retardation, 17,* 59-64.

Cuvo, A. J., & Davis, P. K. (1983). Behavior therapy and community living skills. In M. Herson, R. M. Eisler, & P. M. Miller (Eds.), *Progress in behavior modification, Vol. 4* (pp. 125-172), New York: Academic Press.

Dear, M. (1977). Impact of mental health facilities on property values. *Community Mental Health Journal, 24,* 153-157.

Developmentally Disabled Assistance and Bill of Rights Act of 1975. Public Law 94-103, 42 U.S.C. 6000 et. seq. 89 Stat. 486.

Dunn, L. M. (1968). Special education for the mentally retarded: Is much of it justifiable? *Exceptional Children, 35,* 5-22.

Dunn, L. M. (1973). *Exceptional children in the schools: Special education in transition* (2nd ed.). New York: Rinehart, Holt & Winston.

Education for All Handicapped Children Act of 1975. Public Law 94-142, 20 U.S.C. 1401 et. seq., 89 Stat. 773.

Eyman, R. K., Silverstein, A. B., McLain, R., & Miller, C. (1977). Effects of residential settings on development. In P. Mittler (Ed.), *Research to practice in mental retardation: Care and intervention* (pp. 305-314), Baltimore, MD: University Park Press.

George, M. J., & Baumeister, A. A. (1981). Employee withdrawal and job satisfaction in community residential facilities for mentally retarded persons. *American Journal of Mental Deficiency, 85,* 639-647.

Getzels, J. W., & Guba, E. G. (1957). Social behavior and the administrative process. *School Review, 65,* 423-444.

Getzels, J. W., Lipham, J. M., & Campbell, R. F. (1968). *Educational administration as a social process.* New York: Harper & Row.

Giradeau, F. L., & Spradlin, J. E. (1964). Token rewards in a cottage program. *Mental Retardation, 2*, 345-351.

Goldstein, H., Moss, J. W., & Jordan, L. J. (1965). *The efficacy of special class training on the development of mentally retarded children*. Urbana, IL: University of Illinois. Institute for Research on Exceptional Children.

Gollay, E., Freedman, R., Wyngaarden, M., & Kurtz, N. R. (1978). *Coming back: The community experiences of deinstitutionalized mentally retarded people*. Cambridge, MA: About Books.

Hage, J. (1980). *Theories of organizations: Form, process and transformation*. New York: John Wiley & Sons.

Halderman vs. Pennhurst, 446 F supp. 1295 (1977).

Hendrix, E. (1981). The fallacies in the concept of normalization. *Mental Retardation, 19*, 295-296.

Hewett, F. M., & Forness, S. R. (1974). *Education of exceptional learners*. Boston: Allyn & Bacon.

Hill, J., & Wehman, P. (1980). An initial assessment of the parental needs of severely and profoundly handicapped youth. In P. Wehman & M. Hill (Eds.), *Vocational training and placement of severely disabled persons: Project Employability* (Vol. 2). Richmond, VA: Virginia Commonwealth University State School and Hospital.

Holland, T. (1973). Organizational structure and institutional care. *Journal of Health and Social Behavior, 14*, 241-251.

Itard, J. M. G. (1962). *The wild boy of Aveyron*. New York: Appleton, Prentice-Hall.

Jackson, J. (1969). Factors in the treatment of environment. *Archives of General Psychiatry, 21*, 39-45.

Jacobson, J. W., & Schwartz, A. A. (1983). The evaluation of community living alternatives for developmentally disabled persons. In J. L. Matson & J. A. Mulick (Eds.), *Handbook of mental retardation* (pp. 39-66), New York: Pergamon Press.

Jones, M. L., Risley, T. R., & Favell, J. E. (1983). Ecological patterns. In J. L. Matson & S. E. Bruening (Eds.), *Assessing the mentally retarded* (pp. 311-334), New York: Grune & Stratton.

Kanter, R. M. (1977). *Men and women of the corporation*. New York: Basic Books.

Kastner, L. S., Repucci, N. D., & Pezzoli, J. J. (1979). Assessing community attitudes toward mentally retarded persons. *American Journal of Mental Deficiency, 84*, 137-144.

Kauffman, J. M., & Payne, J. S. (1975). *Mental retardation: Introduction and personal perspectives*. Columbus, OH: Merrill.

Kazdin, A. E. (1982). *Single case research designs: Methods for clinical and applied settings*. New York: Oxford University Press.

Kearly, P. (1984). *The relationship of organizational structural characteristics to modes of conflict management employed by Michigan administrators of special education*. Unpublished doctoral dissertation. Michigan State University, East Lansing, Michigan.

Kimberly, J. R. (1976). Organizational size and the structuralist perspective: A review, critique and proposal. *Administrative Science Quarterly, 21*, 571-597.

King, R. D., Raynes, N. V., & Tizard, J. (1971). *Patterns of residential care: Sociological studies in situations for handicapped citizens*. London: Routledge & Kegan Paul.

Kolstoe, O. P., & Frey, R. M. (1965). *A high school work study program for mentally subnormal students*. Carbondale, IL: Southern Illinois University Press.

Lakin, K. C., Bruininks, R. H., & Sigford, B. B. (1981). Deinstitutionalization and community adjustment: A summary of research and issues. In R. H. Bruininks, C. E. Meyers, B. B. Sigford & K. C. Lakin (Eds.), *Deinstitutionalization and community adjustment of mentally retarded people*. Washington, DC: American Association on Mental Deficiency.

Landesman-Dwyer, S., Sackett, G. P., & Kleinman, J. S. (1980). Relationship of size to resident and staff behavior in small community residences. *American Journal of Mental Deficiency, 85*, 6-17.

Lauber, D., & Bangs, F. S., Jr. (1974). *Zoning for family and group care facilities*. (ASPO, Planning Advisory Service Report No. 300.) Chicago, IL: American Society of Planning Officials.

Lindsley, O. R. (1956). Operant conditioning methods applied to research in chronic schizophrenia. *Psychiatric Research Reports, 5*, 118-139.

Lindsley, O. R. (1960). *Characteristics of the behavior of chronic psychotics as revealed by free-operant conditioning methods*. Discussions of the nervous system. Monograph Supplement, *21*, 66-78.

MacEachron, A. E., & Driscoll, J. W. (1981). *Organizational redesign of physical structure, quality of worklife and performance: A field experience in the human services*. Hiller School Working Paper, Waltham, MA: Brandeis University.

MacMillan, D. L., Jones, R. L., & Aloia, G. F. (1974). The mentally retarded label: A review of research and theoretical analysis. *American Journal of Mental Deficiency, 79*, 241-261.

Mamula, R. A., & Newman, N. (1973). *Community placement of the mentally retarded. A handbook for community agencies and social work practitioners*. Springfield, IL: Thomas.

Marchetti, A., & Matson, J. L. (1981). Training skills for community adjustment. In J. L. Matson & J. R. McCartney (Eds.), *Handbook of behavior modification with the mentally retarded* (pp. 211-246). New York: Plenum Press.

Margolis, J., & Charitonidis, T. (1981). Public reactions to housing for the mentally retarded. *Exceptional Children, 48*, 68-69.

Matson, J. L. (1980). A controlled group study of pedestrian skill training for the mentally retarded. *Behavior Research and Therapy, 18*, 99-106.

McCarver, R. B., & Cavalier, A. R. (1983). Philosophical concepts and attitudes underlying programming for the mentally retarded. In J. L. Matson & F. Andrasik (Eds.), *Treatment Issues and Innovations in Mental Retardation* (pp. 1-31). New York: Plenum Press.

Mercer, J. R. (1973). *Labelling the mentally retarded*. Berkeley: University of California Press.

Mesibov, G. B. (1976). Alternatives to the principle of normalization. *Mental Retardation, 14*, 30-32.

Meyer, R. J. (1980). Attitudes of parents of institutionalized mentally retarded individuals toward deinstitutionalization. *American Journal of Mental Deficiency, 85*, 184-187.

Miller, M. (1974). A review of the principle of normalization in human services by Wolf Wolfensberger. *American Journal of Mental Deficiency, 78*, 505-506.

Moos, R. M. (1975). *Evaluating correctional and community settings*, New York: Wiley.

Morris, R. J., & Brown, D. K. (1983). Legal and ethical issues in behavior modification with mentally retarded persons. In J. L. Matson & F. Andrasik (Eds.), *Treatment issues and innovations in mental retardation* (pp. 61-95). New York: Plenum Press.

National Association for Retarded Citizens (1975). Guidelines for the use of behavioral procedures in state programs for retarded persons. *Mental Retardation Research, 1*, 1-71.

National Association for Retarded Citizens vs. Carey, 466, F. Supp. 610 (E.D.N.Y., 1978).

Neef, N. A., Iwata, B., & Page, T. (1978). Public transportation training: In vivo versus classroom instruction. *Journal of Applied Behavior Analysis, 11*, 331-344.

Nirhira, K., Mink, I. I., & Meyers, E. (1984). Salient dimensions of home environment relevant to child development. In N. R. Ellis & N. W. Brady (Eds.), *International review of research in mental retardation* Vol. 12 (pp. 95-122), Orlando, FL: Academic Press.

Nirje, B. (1969). The normalization principle and its human management implications. In R. B. Kogel & W. Wolfensberger (Eds.), *Changing patterns in residential services for the mentally retarded*, Washington, DC: President's Committee on Mental Retardation.

Novak, A. R., & Berkeley, T. R. (1984). A systems theory approach to deinstitutionalization policies and research. In N. R. Ellis & N. W. Brady (Eds.), *International review of research in mental retardation*, Volume 12 (pp. 245-283), Orlando, FL: Academic Press.

O'Connor, G. (1976). *Home is a good place: A national perspective of community residential facilities for developmentally disabled persons*. (Monograph No. 2). Washington, DC: American Association for Mental Deficiency.

O'Donnell, C. R. (1977). Behavior modification in community settings. In M. Herson, R. M. Eisler, & P. M. Miller (Eds.), *Progress in behavior modification*, Vol. 4 (pp. 69-117), New York: Academic Press.

Okolo, C., & Guskin, S. (1984). Community attitudes toward community placement of mentally retarded persons. In M. R. Ellis & N. W. Bray, *International review of research in mental retardation,* Vol. 12 (pp. 25-66), New York: Academic Press.

Pennings, J. (1973). Measures of organizational structure: A methodological note. *American Journal of Sociology, 79,* 686-704.

Pratt, M. W., Luszcz, M. A., & Brown, M. E. (1980). Measuring dimensions of the quality of care in small community residences. *American Journal of Mental Deficiency, 85,* 188-194.

President's Committee on Mental Retardation (1975). *Gallop Poll shows attitudes on mental retardation improving.* President's Committee on Mental Retardation Message.

President's Panel on Mental Retardation (1962). *Report of the mission to the Netherlands.* Washington, DC: U.S. Government Printing Office.

Pugh, D. S., Hickson, D. J., & Hinings, C. R. (1969). An empirical taxonomy of work organizations. *Administrative Science Quarterly, 14,* 115-126.

Pugh, D. S., Hickson, D. J., Hinings, C. R., & Turner, C. (1968). Dimensions of organizational structure. *Administrative Science Quarterly, 13,* 65-105.

Rhoades, C., & Browning, P. (1977). Normalization at what price? *Mental Retardation, 15,* 24.

Rhodes, W. E. (1975). *A study of child variance: The future.* (Vol. 4). Ann Arbor: The University of Michigan.

Roos, P. (1972). Reconciling behavior modification procedures with the normalization principle. In W. Wolfensberger (Ed.), *The principle of normalization in human services.* Toronto: National Institute on Mental Retardation.

Roos, P. (1974). Human rights and behavior modification. *Mental Retardation, 12,* 3-6.

Rusch, F. R., Connis, R. T., & Sowers (1979). The modification and maintenance of time spent attending to task using social reinforcement, token reinforcement and response cost in an applied restaurant setting. *Journal of Special Education Technology, 2,* 18-26.

Rusch, F. R., & Kazdin, A. E. (1981). Toward a methodology of withdrawal designs for the assessment of response maintenance. *Journal of Applied Behavior Analysis, 14,* 131-140.

Schalock, R. L., Harper, R. S., & Carver, G. (1981). Independent living placement: Five years later. *American Journal of Mental Deficiency, 86,* 170-177.

Scheerenberger, R. C. (1978). Public residential services for the mentally retarded. In N. Ellis (Ed.), *International review of research on mental retardation* (Vol. 9). New York Academic Press.

Schinke, S., & Wong, S. (1977). Evaluation of staff training in group homes for retarded persons. *American Journal of Mental Deficiency, 82,* 130-136.

Scott, W. R. (1981). *Organizations: rational, natural and open systems.* Englewood Cliffs, NJ: Prentice-Hall.

Segal, S. P., & Aviram, U. (1978). *The mentally ill and community-based sheltered care.* New York: Wiley.

Sitkei, E. G. (1980). After group home living—what alternatives? Results of a two year mobility follow-up study. *Mental Retardation, 18,* 9-13.

Skinner, B. F. (1938). *The behavior of organisms: An experimental analysis.* New York: Appleton Century.

Smith, F. (1981). *Community acceptance of homes for mentally retarded people.* Unpublished doctoral dissertation, Ann Arbor: University of Michigan.

Thompson, T., & Wray, L. (1985). A behavior analytic approach to community integration of persons with developmental disabilities. In K. C. Lakin & R. H. Bruininks (Eds.), *Strategies for achieving community integration of developmentally disabled citizens.* Baltimore: Brookes, 1985.

Throne, J. M. (1975). The normalization principle: Right ends, wrong means. *Mental Retardation, 13,* 23-25.

Throne, J. M. (1979). Deinstitutionalization: Too wide a swath. *Mental Retardation, 17,* 171-175.

Trippi, J., Michael, R., Colao, A., & Alverez, A. (1978). Housing discrimination toward mentally retarded persons. *Exceptional Children, 44,* 430-437.

VandePol, R. A., Iwata, B. A., Ivancic, M. T., Page, T. J., Neef, N. A., & Whitley, F. P. (1981). Teaching the handicapped to eat in public places: Acquisition generalization and maintenance of restaurant skills. *Journal of Applied Behavior Analysis, 14,* 61-69.

Vincent, L. J., Salisburg, C., Walter, G., Brown, P., Grunewald, L. J., & Powers, M. (1980). Program evaluation and curriculum development in early childhood special education: Criteria for the next environment. In W. Sailor, B. Wilcox, & L. Brown (Eds.), *Methods of instruction for severely handicapped students,* Baltimore: Brookes.

Vogelsburg, R. T., & Rusch, F. R. (1979). Training severely handicapped students to cross partially controlled intersections. *AAESPH Review, 4,* 264-273.

Weick (1976). Educational organizations as loosely coupled systems. *Administrative Science Quarterly, 21,* 1-11.

Weiner, D., Anderson, R. J., & Nietupski, J. (1982). Impact of community-based residential facilities for mentally retarded adults on surrounding property values using a realtor analysis method. *Education and Training of the Mentally Retarded, 17,* 278-282.

Willms, J. D. (1978). *Retarded adults in the community: An investigation of neighborhood attitudes and concerns.* Bethesda, MD: ERIC Document Reproduction Service No. Ed. 162-474.

Wolf, M. (1978). Social Validity or how applied behavior analysis is finding its heart. *Journal of Applied Behavior Analysis, 11,* 203-214.

Wolfensberger, W. (1972). *The principle of normalization in human services.* Toronto: National Institute on Mental Retardation.

Wolfensberger, W. (1980). The definition of normalization: Update problems, disagreements and misunderstanding. In R. J. Flynn & K. Enitsch (Eds.), *Normalization, social integration, and community services.* Baltimore: University Park Press, 19-54.

Wolfensberger, W., & Glenn, L. (1975). PASS 3: Program analysis of service systems: Field Manual. Toronto: National Institute on Mental Retardation.

Wyatt vs. Ireland Civil Action #3195-N, unreported (M.D. Ala. October, 25, 1979).

Wyatt vs. Stickney, 325. F supp. 781 (M.D. Ala (1971), 344 F supp. 1341 (M.D. Ala 1971), 344 F supp. 373, 387 (M.D. Ala, 1972) aff'd in part, modified in part sub norm., Wyatt vs. Vanderholt, 503 F. 2nd. 1305 (th Cir. 1974).

Zeaman, D., House, B. J., & Orlando, R. (1958). Use of special training conditions in the visual discrimination learning with imbeciles. *American Journal of Mental Deficiency, 63,* 453-459.

SECTION II:
ISSUES IN ASSESSMENT
AND TRAINING

Measurement of Adaptive Behavior: Origins, Trends, Issues

Howard G. Cohen

ABSTRACT. Recent legislation and litigation have focused considerable clinical attention on the social integration of people with handicaps into the community mainstream. Measures of adaptive behavior have played an increasingly important part in this endeavor. They serve two primary functions: classification/placement and program planning/treatment. This paper traces the conceptual origins of adaptive behavior from state residential institutions to its role in the complex process of community integration. A framework for evaluating and selecting adaptive behavior scales is presented along with a review of current trends in measurement. The last section discusses conceptual and methodological issues that presently confront the adaptive behavior field.

The demand for ways to measure adaptive behavior has recently escalated dramatically. Spreat, Roszkowski and Isett (1983) estimate that well over 200 instruments purporting to measure adaptive behavior have emerged in the last 20 years. Many of these are "home grown," target specific populations (e.g., severely to profoundly mentally retarded), have limited utility, and do not meet even minimal technical standards for assessment instruments (Meyers, Nihira, & Zetlin, 1979). Yet, legislation and litigation, primarily in the 1970s, fueled by sweeping changes in public attitudes toward treatment of individuals with handicaps, have literally compelled the usage of adaptive behavior scales in the school, community, residential institution, and other treatment settings. Choosing from among such a wide variety of existing adaptive behavior tools

Howard G. Cohen is affiliated with the Valley Mountain Regional Center, 701 Dundee Way, Stockton, CA 95210.

or, alternatively, deciding to create one to meet unique requirements of a treatment setting can be a confusing and overwhelming task.

The purpose of this chapter is two-fold: (a) to develop a framework for understanding the concept of adaptive behavior as it has evolved and is currently applied in the diagnosis and treatment of individuals with handicaps and (b) to provide technical assistance in making sound selections of instruments to measure adaptive behavior. The chapter will be divided into two major sections.

The first part will review significant sociopolitical forces that have propelled adaptive behavior to the forefront and focus on assessment and habilitation efforts with handicapped individuals. The conceptual foundations of adaptive behavior and attempts to quantify and measure it will be delineated. Its origins in state residential institutions for the mentally retarded from the middle 1930s to the 1960s will be reviewed. A discussion of the ascendancy and refinement of adaptive behavior instruments during the deinstitutionalization era of the 1960s and 1970s will follow. The second section will focus on three topics: presentation of a systematic method to match adaptive behavior instrument selection with user function, review of six emergent trends in adaptive behavior assessment, and discussion about the conceptual and methodological roadblocks adaptive behavior measures must overcome to become viable assessment tools for the future.

It is not the intent of this chapter to provide an all-inclusive compendium of commercially available adaptive behavior measures (see Walls, Werner, Bacon, & Zane, 1977; Coulter & Morrow, 1978; Mayeda, Pelzer, & Van Zuylen, 1978; Meyers et al., 1979). Rather, this chapter will focus on adaptive behavior measures that either have made a significant conceptual contribution to the field or reflect current and future national trends in adaptive behavior usage.

CONCEPTUAL FOUNDATIONS

Every culture and subculture establishes minimum standards of acceptable behavior for its members. Adaptive behavior or social competence is conceptualized as the perceived fit between individual performance and societal expectations at any one point in time. Performance standards are not universal, but are culture and chronological age-specific. Expectations for eight-year-olds growing up in Kansas City and Peking certainly differ. Additionally, children from both of these diverse cultures are not required to meet the performance expectations of their teen and adult counterparts. The individual's capacity to adapt or fit is often determined by peer/public perceptions and attitudes, and not necessarily by actual behavior. For example, earlier in this century, an individual labeled mentally deficient was perceived as unfit or maladaptive solely on the basis of an intelligence quotient (IQ).

Measurement of adaptive behavior involves two sequential processes. First, an attempt is made to identify and quantify a social system's behavior standards or expectations. For example, Heber (1961) argued that societal expectations for adults living within the mainstream of American culture included minimally the ability for self-maintenance and personal-social responsibility. Second, a methodology is developed to evaluate individual performance against those standards. This linkage between theory building (i.e., What is adaptive behavior?) and scale development will be explored in this section.

The measurement of adaptive behavior serves two primary functions. First, the data can be used to identify, classify, and diagnose individuals along a dimension of perceived social competency-incompetency. A child's relative position on this continuum can be used to guide, for example, decisions about special education placement. Second, adaptive behavior data can be used to plan and evaluate treatment and intervention strategies. More often than not, the classification function is primary and dictates the range of intervention options available.

Historically, social and political attitudes have determined the actual dimensions upon which to measure adaptive behavior. Wolfensberger (1976) has traced the history of various classification schemes and their subsequent impact on the treatment of handicapped individuals. These effects have included outcasting, isolation, protection, and even death. A prevailing attitude toward handicapped in the first two-thirds of this century was that of an immutable, but relatively harmless, social incompetent (Sarason & Doris, 1969). This societal attitude of a permanent adaptive disability was reinforced by the intelligence testing movement and by early findings in developmental psychology. The product of the testing movement became the Intelligence Quotient (IQ). The scientific community's endorsement of the IQ was given on the basis that it was found to be reliable, stable over time, and could predict certain future achievements (e.g., academic success). The broader concept of social competence was lost, and subsequently, capability was represented by scores on tests of intelligence (Mercer, 1978). Behavior in a standardized testing situation was characterized as representative of the individual's total social adaptation. Scores on IQ tests increasingly became the sole criteria upon which diagnosis, placements, and treatment decisions were made (Mercer, 1973).

During this same era, developmentalists such as Gesell and Amatruda (1941) and Piaget (1952) identified uniform developmental sequences or stages. An individual's achievement at any one point in time, it was reasoned, could be catalogued along this developmental dimension. Utilization of these scales to represent levels of achievement such as mental age (Terman, 1916), developmental age (Gesell & Amatruda, 1941), and social age (Doll, 1953) gained prominence. There was an implicit assumption during this time that regardless of chronological age, an individual's social functioning could be reduced to a fixed point on a developmental continuum. Therefore, levels of adaptive behavior could be represented by a score on an IQ test or a mental age equivalent. Adaptive behavior became associated with a more or less stable and permanent condition of an individual. A logical treatment strategy stemming from this conception involved concentrating on the care, protection, and isolation of individuals who fell into this category. In response, there was an unprecedented expansion of large public residential facilities for the mentally retarded in the United States (Kugel & Shearer, 1976). By 1967, the number of institutionalized children and adults labeled mentally retarded approached 200,000 nationwide (Butterfield, 1976).

In the last 25 years, there has been a dramatic change in public attitude and political action toward individuals with handicaps. These changes have led to a reconceptualization of adaptive behavior and to radically altered treatment strategies. Four factors fueling this shift in attitude will be discussed. First, deleterious effects of institutionalization were brought to public attention in dramatic fashion by articles such as Wolfensberger's (1969) *Origin and Nature of Our Institutional Models* and by pictorial essays such as Blatt and Kaplan's (1966) *Christmas in Purgatory*. Second, the President's Committee on Mental Retardation (1969, 1976) published a highly influential compendium of articles, promulgating the adoption of the philosophy of *normalization* to service delivery and offering alternative community-based models. Residential treatment models based on the principle of normalization had already gained wide recognition in the Scandinavian countries but were, at that time, relatively unknown in the United States. Nirje (1976) defined normalization as a process by which all people, including handicapped people, have equal opportunity to participate in the regular pattern and conditions of everyday life.

Changes in public perceptions about the mentally retarded led to the deinstitutionalization movement (Bruininks, Thurlow, Thurman, & Fiorelli, 1980) and to a reformulation of the developmental model. That is, attention shifted toward day-to-day activities that people need in the community to take care of personal needs, to get around, to get along with others, and to become economically self-sufficient. Butterfield (1976) reported a study conducted by the Social Security Administration which found that admissions to institutions were most commonly based on *skill deficits* and *behavior maladjustment* in the community. That is, individuals were initially identified for institutionalization, not by their low scores on IQ tests, but much more commonly by their perceived inability to perform the critical personal and social skills expected for individuals of their age and from their community. While developmental sequences were believed to remain orderly and predictable, the rate and progression of development was perceived as modifiable. The concept of the IQ began to be seen as separate or distinct from that of adaptive behavior in at least two ways. First, the IQ, because of its perceived stability and emphasis on language, reasoning and abstract abilities (Grossman, 1983), was seen as being of very little help in guiding the acquisition of more basic concrete daily living skills. Second, the IQ was seen as evaluating the potential for performance rather than typical performance.

Wide-ranging legislation and litigation in the 1970s catapulted adaptive behavior measurement from use as a scientific construct to a primary place in decision-making regarding nondiscriminatory evaluation, educational placement, appropriate education, and least restrictive placement (Boone, 1983). For example, PL 94-142, The Education for All Handicapped Children Act of 1975, specifies that multiple assessment sources, including adaptive behavior measures, must be used prior to placing a child in a more restrictive educational placement (Martin, 1979). Court cases such as Diana vs. State Board of Education (1970) and Larry P. vs. Riles (1972) significantly altered testing practices (Turnbull & Turnbull, 1979). The common practice of using IQ test scores as the sole basis for educational placement was now labeled as racially discriminatory. Instead, the courts mandated that placement decisions be based on the child's culturally-based learning and experiences. Adaptive behavior, of course, was seen as yielding the kind of information that was compatible with the court decisions.

A fourth factor that gave adaptive behavior measures a high profile centered on changes in clinical practice of diagnosis and classification of mental retardation. Heber (1959, 1961) introduced the concept of adaptive behavior into the American Association of Mental Deficiency (AAMD) classification scheme of mental retardation. Mental retardation was defined as an impairment in intellectual functioning associated with deficits in adaptive behavior. Grossman (1973) made it explicit that *concurrent* deficits in intellectual and adaptive functioning must be present in order to make a clinically proper diagnosis of mental retardation. Up until that time there was a clinical presumption that intelligence tests were able to measure a general ability and social competence. Despite the establishment of adaptive behavior as an independent dimension of mental retardation, controversy around such fundamental issues as definition, administrative procedures, standardization, reliability, validity, and relationship to intelligence remain strong issues (Coulter & Morrow, 1978b). Nevertheless, there is a present consensus among major classification manuals American Psychiatric Association, 1980; International Classification of Diseases, 1980; AAMD Classification Manual in Mental Retardation, Grossman, 1983) that endorses the concurrent evaluation of both intelligence and adaptive behavior before making a diagnosis of mental retardation. In fact, Leland (1972) has suggested that adaptive behavior may be a reasonable alternative to IQ testing.

In summary, particularly since 1970, changes in the philosophy of the treatment of handicapped, emphasis on community integration, legislation, litigation, and changes in clinical practice mandated that adaptive behavior measures, although ill-equipped conceptually and technically, be employed in the diagnosis, placement, program planning, training, and intervention of individuals with handicaps. The application of adaptive behavior to these issues brought with it hopes and dreams of reversing the isolating and segregating effects of severe intellectual deficit.

ORIGINS OF ADAPTIVE BEHAVIOR (AB) MEASUREMENT

The purpose of initial attempts to define and measure adaptive behavior was tied to the acquisition of desirable behaviors among children and adults living in institutions for the mentally retarded (Morrow & Coulter, 1978). The IQ was well entrenched and controlled much of the diagnostic and placement process. Yet, many of those working directly with the residents of institutions recognized that the IQ yielded little useful information about an individual's day-to-day performance. Pioneers in the assessment of adaptive behavior were primarily concerned with establishing adaptive behavior as an independent dimension. Their focus of attention was to identify, measure, and then to remediate perceived social deficits (Leland, 1973). Most of the AB measures that will be cited in this section are still in wide use. But, it is not their ability to endure that is relevant. Each represents a struggle to operationalize diverse theoretical notions about what adaptive behavior is and how it can be measured. These original attempts at measuring adaptive behavior began to lay out the parameters for a definition of social competency.

Vineland Social Maturity Scale (VSMS)

Doll (1953) can be considered the "father" of the 20th century adaptive behavior assessment field. Working at the Training School at Vineland, New Jersey, he published the first edition of the Vineland Social Maturity Scale (VSMS) in 1936. Doll was looking for a tool that would measure increases in a resident's "social useful-ness" (Doll, 1953, p.4) as a result of exposure to various training techniques. He defined social competence as the "functional ability of the human organism for exercising personal independence and social responsibility" (Doll, 1953, p.10). In his pioneering work on adaptive behavior, he set the tone for future inquiry by establishing the following: (a) social competence refers to the progressive devel-opment or maturation of the human organism; (b) adaptive behavior can be quantified by sampling representative performance at suc-cessive age levels, expressed in social age (SA) units; (c) adaptive behavior differs from measures of intelligence in that it samples actual day-to-day performance of basic living skills rather than in-nate or perceived intellectual or academic abilities; (d) adaptive be-havior scales must not only yield a measure of total competence, which he expressed as a social quotient (SQ), but also must provide a description or analysis of the components of competence; and (e) reliable data about an individual can be gathered by interviewing a third party informant (e.g., parent, primary care provider, teacher) rather than through direct observation or by formalized testing.

To establish norms for his scale, Doll gathered data on 620 sub-jects living in a semi-rural community that surrounded the Vineland School locale. He divided the sample into 31 year-groupings from birth to 30 years. The age of achievement was computed for each item on the original scale. It is important to note that while the application was conceived in terms of the institution, the actual data upon which the scale was based was taken from a community sam-ple.

The VSMS (1953) in current use consists of 117 statements about the performance of skills, divided into 17 age periods. The items generally tap two types of skills: skills that lead toward personal independence and skills that lead toward social responsibility. Per-sonal independence includes skill categories such as self-help, com-munication, and locomotion. Social responsibility includes skill categories such as self-direction, socialization, and occupation. Doll's intent was to develop a scale that could be useful in training and evaluating the effects of training. However, primarily because of his attempt to establish nonhandicapped reference norms, it has enjoyed wide use by clinicians as an AB instrument useful in the classification and diagnosis of mental retardation.

Although Heber (1961) did not develop a formal AB measurement tool, he contributed significantly to the development of a construct of adaptive behavior. Prior to 1970, there were few commercially available AB tools. Informal assessment was, much of the time, the primary means of gaining insight into the day-to-day skill performance of individuals. Heber (1961) and Grossman (1973) proposed adaptive behavior parameters that became useful in this type of evaluation. Heber defined adaptive behavior as the effectiveness with which an individual copes with the physical and social demands of his culture. According to Heber, impairments in adaptive behavior could be manifested in three areas of development: maturation, learning, and social adjustment. Each of these areas takes on differential importance relative to a person's chronological age. Maturation is critical in early childhood development.

Deficits in maturation are manifested by delays or inability to achieve mastery of developmental milestones (e.g., walking, talking, toileting, etc.). Deficits in learning (e.g., reading, writing, math) become crucial during the school-age years. Deficits in social adjustment in adulthood relate more to an inability to develop and maintain personal independence and gainful employment. Grossman cited guidelines in the AAMD Classification Manual (1973) that expanded Heber's description. He then correlated adaptive behavior achievement levels with chronological age expectations and degree of severity of mental retardation. The adaptive behavior constructs formulated by Heber and Grossman contributed to a systematic method for observing the concrete behavioral patterns of individuals with handicaps.

AAMD Adaptive Behavior Scale (ABS)

In 1965, the American Association on Mental Deficiency sponsored a project at Parsons State Hospital in Kansas to build a more comprehensive definition of adaptive behavior and to evolve a measurement tool based on this definition (Leland, 1973; Coulter & Morrow, 1978b). Leland (1973) introduced two key concepts which would guide the development of an adaptive behavior assessment tool through the Parsons Project. First, he argued that minimum social competency can be described as a form of *invisibility*. He felt that mentally retarded people were typically identified and earmarked for institutionalization not by cognitive deficiencies, but as a result of the manifestation of visible deviant behavior that brings them to the attention of the community. He suggested that the primary need is to identify critical behaviors (e.g., public manners) that maintain this invisibility. Once those behaviors were identified, the task would be to systematically teach them to the residents of the institution. When these skills are acquired, residents could return to the mainstream community, thereby *reversing* the process. Leland believed that the behavior technology was already available to build personal and social skills to assist the individual in blending in and to eliminate maladaptive behaviors that might interfere with this integration.

Leland outlines three parameters of adaptive behavior: independent functioning, personal responsibility, and social responsibility. Independent functioning is similar to Doll's concept of social maturation. It follows a sequential pattern of emergence around the acquisition of basic living skills considered necessary to function in our culture (e.g., personal hygiene, mobility around the community, money handling, survival reading, etc.). Personal responsibility taps the individual's motivation to take on responsibility for her own actions. This revolves around the person's ability to make conscious rational choices and to resist exploitation. Social responsibility taps the individual's responsiveness and awareness of behavior expected from individuals in her age group and culture. This could range from probing the person's understanding of and compliance with laws regulating criminal conduct (e.g., crossing busy intersections, stealing); to evaluating the ability of the individual to exercise control over maladaptive habits or emotions (e.g., picking nose in public, interpersonal aggressiveness). Leland stresses that performance of personal and social responsibilities are key components of adult social competence.

The AAMD Adaptive Behavior Scale (ABS) (Nihira, Foster, Shellhaas, & Leland, 1974) emerged as the instrument from this conceptual base and research project. It consists of two major parts. Part I consists of 10 domains involving basic adaptive skills; Part II consists of 14 domains that tap maladaptive behaviors. Norms are available. Percentiles were derived for each of the 24 domains on 11 age groups from ages three to 69 based on a sampling of 200 institutionalized residents at each age group. Empirical support for this approach was provided by factor analysis of raw and domain scores (Nihira, 1978). Three factor clusters were found: personal self-sufficiency, community self-sufficiency, and personal-social responsibility.

The development of the ABS has made a number of significant contributions to the field of adaptive behavior measurement. First, remediation and treatment became the primary outcome objectives of AB assessment. Data interpretation focusing on domain cluster scores (Leland, 1978), rather than on a general or overall score, reinforced this notion. It fostered the idea that adaptive behavior is not an immutable trait, but rather a constellation of specific strengths and weaknesses of an individual. Specific deficits are targeted for reversal and remediation through behavioral training procedures. Second, the ABS provided the foundation for a functional habilitation model. It veers away from the notion implicit in the VSMS that social competence is exclusively tied to a fixed maturational progression. For example, a 12-year-old adolescent may achieve a social age of five on the VSMS. Using the developmental model, the trainer's task would focus on increasing this person's social age to six, seven or even eight. In contrast, the ABS emphasizes attainment of skills that foster higher levels of functional independence. For example, increasing reading skills from a first grade level to a third or fourth grade level is seen as less important than achievement of a survival word recognition level that would allow the person to identify the correct bus to a specific destination, thereby increasing independent mobility around the community. Third, the ABS's inclusion of maladaptive behavior domains such as antisocial behavior, withdrawal, and odd mannerisms demonstrate that these are also critical aspects of adaptive behavior that need to be identified and remediated as well.

Progress Assessment Chart (P-A-C)

Gunzburg (1973, 1976) developed the Progress Assessment Chart (P-A-C) in Britain, but it has enjoyed wide use in the United States through its USA-Indiana distributor, Aux Chandelles. Gunzburg postulated that the demands and customs of a community are so bewildering to the mentally retarded child that a weakened personality structure develops that leads to underachievement. Gunzburg reasoned that a systematic training and educational program emphasizing pragmatic living skills and the design of natural environments that foster learning is vital. This can lead to a reactivation of personal motivation toward social competence and achievement of acceptability in the community (Gunzburg, 1976). The P-A-C was developed by Gunzburg to measure the success of these efforts. It was designed to be a measurement tool that could be repeated often. Results are presented graphically and quantitatively to quickly gauge success or failure of training.

The P-A-C consists of six separate forms: P-P-A-C for profoundly retarded children and for children of normal development from birth to three years; the P-A-C I designed for moderately and severely retarded children or normally developing children from six to 16 years of age; the P-A-C II for moderate, mild, and borderline mentally retarded older adolescents and adults; the P-A-C IA (an extension of the P-A-C I) for the advanced adolescent; the M/P-A-C I which is aimed specifically at Down's Syndrome children from six to 15 years of age; and the F/P-A-C for young and middle-aged severely handicapped adults. Normed primarily on institutionalized populations, the P-A-C yields an overall social competence index. Four domain scores are available relative to age and IQ level: self-help, communication, socialization, and occupation. Individual items are arranged in ascending concentric rings called a psychogram. As scores progress to the outer rings the social usefulness and complexity of the individual is assumed to be more advanced.

Reliability and validity information are absent in the manual. Similar to the VSMS, detailed instructions are available in the manual to guide the rater. Even though some of the items are peculiar to the British population, the P-A-C is popular in the United States because the items are well-defined behaviorally and appear to relate well to the kinds of skills necessary for people to live in the community.

Balthazar Scales

Balthazar (1971, 1973) deserves mention as a pioneer. His work with severely and profoundly mentally retarded residents at Central Wisconsin Colony and Training School (Central Wisconsin Center for the Developmentally Disabled) produced two scales: Scales of Functional Independence and the Scales of Social Adaptation. His approach was distinguished in two important ways from previous research literature. First, he tirelessly collected data by observing actual behavior of residents on the wards to develop the content and sequencing of items for his AB scales. This research method was in contrast to the more commonly used approach that relied either on pre-existing child development data for normal development or on interviews with child development experts. Balthazar did not assume that development for normal and abnormal children was identical. Second, he established direct observational criteria for scoring each item. Balthazar focused his attention equally on rater and ratee. Criticisms of the scale include its narrow content, limited target population and the time needed to complete the scale. However, it remains as an example of the kind of scientific rigor that must be present in order for adaptive behavior measures to meet profession-wide credibility standards.

In summary, the concept of AB measurement was initially conceived and refined within an institutional framework. Definition and design of these tools were specifically oriented to the needs of the institutionalized population (Morrow & Coulter, 1978). They were primarily utilized for training and monitoring basic skills (e.g., self-care) and reducing maladaptive behaviors (e.g., self-stimulation, destructive behaviors). During the 1970s, public interest in the application of AB measurements shifted substantially from the small population of mentally retarded individuals living in state residential institutions to the larger number of handicapped people living in the community. At the same time, interest in the application of AB tools to guide the identification of training objectives and in intervention was supplanted by an increasing interest in classification and placement (e.g., special education placement of the handicapped). Although many of these instruments continued to be used to measure adaptive behavior performance in the community, they had significant shortcomings. While norms may have been available, they were most always inappropriate. The VSMS was normed on a small geographically unrepresentative sample (Song & Jones, 1982) and norms for the ABS were developed from mentally retarded individuals living in institutions. These instruments were ill-prepared for the kind of placement and identification issues that were to become of primary concern in a community-based system. However, one project which originated in the 1950s at Pacific State Hospital in California, studied the transition of handicapped individuals from the institution to the community. This led to an adaptive behavior assessment that was more relevant to these community issues.

Pacific State Hospital Project

In 1954, Pacific State Hospital in California began a series of projects to study the families of mentally retarded individuals living in the community. This led to the development of anthropological and statistical methodology to study the incidence of mental retardation in the community (Dingman, 1973). Mercer (1973) studied the proportion of minority representation in special education classes in the Riverside County school system. IQ was the primary gatekeeper of that system. Results from Mercer's research showed that black and Mexican/American children, as well as children from lower socioeconomic backgrounds, tended to be overrepresented in special education. When dual criteria were used (i.e., IQ and AB measures), children from nonminority and higher socioeconomic strata were underrepresented. Mercer used the term, *six hour child* (President's Committee on Mental Retardation, 1970) to refer to minority children who functioned quite well in the social system outside of school, but who were labeled mentally retarded within the school system, primarily, on the basis of poor academic achievement (Mercer, 1975). This led to a search for an assessment system that would first, ameliorate some of the built-in bias of previous assessment tools and secondly, take into account behavior expectations of the individual's social culture setting. She developed a comprehensive system called the System of Multicultural Pluralistic Assessment (SOMPA). One component within that system is a measure of adaptive behavior, the Adaptive Behavior Inventory for Children (ABIC). This, and Mercer's labeling theory, will be discussed more fully in a later section.

SELECTING AN ADAPTIVE BEHAVIOR (AB) INSTRUMENT

The selection of an AB measurement instrument appropriate to setting and function is made more difficult by the high numbers of tools presently available in the marketplace. To aid in this selection process, differences among AB measures can be analyzed along several critical dimensions. For example, Morrow and Coulter (1978) developed a rating form which provides a structured format for evaluating the usefulness of any AB measure under consideration. Information is gathered on compliance to state-defined standards, instrument content, and administrative considerations (e.g., cost). In this section, a five-step procedure will be outlined to help the prospective consumer of AB instruments make sound selection choices.

Function

Gathering useful adaptive behavior information begins with a clear understanding of purpose. Clarifying the purpose or function for employing an AB measure guides the entire selection process. Adaptive behavior measures serve two primary functions: classification/placement and program planning/training. The following are examples of the first function: differential diagnosis (e.g., borderline functioning vs. mental retardation), eligibility for special programs for the handicapped, allocation of funds for programs at the state level, placement in a more/less restrictive treatment environment, and identification of program needs of one group versus another (e.g., handicapped vs. nonhandicapped). The following are examples of the second function: grouping individuals by skill levels/deficits for intervention purposes, individual program planning, and evaluating/monitoring the progress of an individual/group relative to a criterion (e.g., telephone independence). An instrument that satisfies the criteria for one purpose may not be very useful for another. For example, if placement in special education versus placement in a regular class is an issue, then an AB instrument that has norms comparing an individual's performance to other mentally retarded children may be practically useless.

Instrument Content

Most AB scales cover at least three skill domains: self-help, communication, and socialization (Mayeda et al, 1978). Other domains incorporated vary from instrument to instrument but may include: motor skills, vocational/prevocational skills, travel/mobility, self-responsibility, and maladaptive behavior. Typically, the target individual receives a rating based on degree of independent performance for each item in the scale. Type of ratings include: completeness of task performance, percentage of time the task is self-initiated, and type of assistance necessary to complete task (e.g., physical guidance vs. imitation vs. verbal prompt). Ratings are based on what the individual *does* (i.e., typical performance), and rarely on what he *can* (i.e., optimal performance). The content of a scale can vary in-*band* and in-*depth* of coverage. Band refers to the number of domains covered, ranging from narrow to comprehensive. Depth refers to the extent a domain is probed, ranging from cursory to extensive. A match between scale content and user (consumer) function is crucial. For example, when classification/placement is the most important use of the scale, then band of coverage plays the important role because the score(s) must represent the individual's overall adaptive functioning. When program planning/training is the key parameter, then depth of coverage is of greater concern to the user.

Content considerations should include: Is the scale's band of coverage comprehensive or narrow? Is the scale's depth of coverage cursory or extensive? Are user-relevant skills covered (e.g., monetary skills)? Are domains covered sufficiently (e.g., two scale items vs. ten scale items)? Are school-related and/or out-of-school behaviors emphasized? Are the items in a domain ordered from simple to complex? Does the scale emphasize developmental (e.g., skills that most children attain by the age of three) versus academic (e.g., reading, math) versus functional (e.g., community survival skills)? Are maladaptive skills included (e.g., frequency and severity of hitting, negative self-references, etc.)? Are results reported by domain scores, factor scores, and/or composite scores?

Method of Administration

The method employed by an AB instrument to collect data on individual performance has significant bearing on the interpretation of results. There are two primary methods: direct and indirect. Spreat et al. (1983) further subdivide indirect administration procedures into two categories: interview and third party. In the third party assessment method, the informant, an individual familiar with the client, fills out the scale. Under the interview format a trained specialist obtains information from the informant and fills out the scale concurrently or after the interview.

Two methods have been used to obtain data more directly. For example, Linkenhoker and McCarron (1980) have developed a nonverbal test of community survival skills. Balthazar (1973) has developed both a test and observational method. Direct observational methods are tied so closely to concrete reality that problems with reliability and memory are minimized. However, time considerations and limited sampling of behaviors across settings create difficulty in the widespread clinical application of these methods. Third party assessment is perhaps the weakest method of scale administration. The rater is responsible for understanding what is being asked, how to fill the form out correctly, and extensive familiarity with the client (Spreat et al., 1983). The interview method is probably a good compromise because it pairs an individual familiar with the scale and interview methods with an individual familiar with the target client. Reliability between the informant's perception and the client's actual performance remains a nagging problem.

Factors in method of administration that contribute to the interpretive validity of the test results include: use of standardized instructions, availability of training workshops for users, behavior specificity of scale items, and specific scoring criteria for scale items. For example, in the area of monetary skills, a scale item that merely states *budgets money* is a vague statement and may result in an answer that does not fully elicit what is intended. Alternatively, the scale item *pays bills before they are overdue* is more specific and may lead to a more reliable answer.

Psychometric Characteristics

Knowledge about the technical construction and validation studies undertaken in the development of an AB measure allows the test user to draw conclusions about an individual's test/scale performance. Three psychometric variables will be discussed: norming, reliability, and validity.

Mayeda et al. (1978) surveyed 69 AB measurement tools. Approximately 33% provided data on psychometric properties. In fact, Spreat et al. (1983) speculate that the overall figure is probably substantially less. However, the situation is improving immeasurably in the 1980s. Most of the AB scales that will be reviewed in the next section provide the user with ample technical data.

Norm-referenced scales permit the user to make comparisons between an individual's performance and a specific reference group. Demographic parameters of the reference group may include: age, sex, disability, education, and geographical location. Standardization refers to a methodology whereby statistical data are collected on the reference group to represent a normal distribution of demographic characteristics (i.e., representative of the United States population). This type of norming is called a representative stratified sample. Not all scales that report norms are standardized. The individual's position relative to the comparison group is typically summarized by some or all of the following statistical indices: standard scores (with a mean of 100 and standard deviation of 15), percentiles, stanines, and developmental, or social age equivalencies.

Criterion-referenced measures allow for a comparison between an individual's current performance level and a predetermined standard or criterion. The criterion or standard is arbitrary. It represents the mastery or fulfillment of an objective. For example, the criterion might be represented by the client obtaining a job in the community. A sequence of increasingly complex tasks can be defined as prerequisites to obtaining this objective. Comparisons can be made between a person's present skill level and that of the criterion. Comparisons between the individual's current performance and the standard or criterion is usually expressed in percentage of mastery. For example, the individual has met 60% of the criterion.

AB instruments differ in the type and quality of norms available. Awareness of norms for a particular AB tool better prepares the user to match instrument selection with purpose for use. For example, if diagnosis is a primary purpose for utilizing an AB instrument, then a standardized, norm-referenced scale is preferred. The majority of scales discussed in this chapter are norm-referenced and, therefore, have some utility for diagnostic and placement issues.

Norm-referenced scales can be converted to criterion-referenced scales, but the reverse is not true. However, norm-referenced measures that are useful in screening program eligibility may not be particularly helpful in tracking progress on more fine-grained training objectives. The following chapter deals with the technology of constructing functional criterion-referenced scales.

The reliability and validity of an AB measurement tool are important whether the purpose of the assessment is classification/placement or program planning/intervention. Reliability refers to the consistency of measurement. There are essentially four types of reliability measures: inter-rater, test-retest, internal consistency, and standard error of measurement. With the exception of the standard error of measurement, reliability is expressed in terms of a reliability coefficient. A reliability coefficient ranging from the .80 to .99 is considered satisfactory, meeting the basic reliability standards. Inter-rater reliability refers to the degree of consistency between two or more independent raters. Test-retest reliability refers to the consistency of measurement when the assessment is repeated over a short time. Internal consistency or split-half reliability measures the degree of consistency among the items. The standard error of measurement (SEM) reflects the level of confidence that can be placed on the accuracy of the measurement scores at any one point in time (Meyers et al., 1979).

Validity generally refers to the level of confidence in making inferences about an individual's performance based on test scores

(Standards, 1985). Spreat et al. (1983) discuss two basic approaches to validity. The first approach refers to the accuracy with which the test or scale measures what it purports to measure. Content, construct, and concurrent are typical of the types of validities reported. The second approach is called predictive validity. It indicates the efficiency with which the current scores on the test can predict future performance.

In evaluating the usefulness of an AB instrument, the following psychometric parameters should be considered: (a) Is a chapter or technical supplement available which summarizes test construction, reliability, and validity studies? (b) Is the standard error of measurement (SEM) cited in the technical manual and is it represented on the profile sheet which displays test results? (c) Are reliability coefficients cited and generally in the .80s range and above? (d) Are norms cited? How are they expressed (e.g., standard scores, percentiles, age equivalents)? Do norms match intended purpose?

Administrative Considerations

A final consideration in the selection of an appropriate AB instrument centers on some administrative concerns. First, what is the cost of purchasing the basic assessment materials and the subsequent costs of reordering record or profile forms? Second, how much time is needed to administer the test, score the test, and communicate the test results? For example, some of the recently published AB instruments give the user the option of computer scoring which can save considerable time. Third, what is the cost and time that is necessary to train personnel how to administer, score, and interpret the assessment instrument?

CURRENT TRENDS IN ADAPTIVE BEHAVIOR MEASUREMENT

Six current approaches to the measurement of adaptive behavior are reviewed in this section. Three criteria were used as a basis to screen AB instruments that represent each approach. First, because the actual content areas or domains covered by an AB scale can be so diverse, the authors of the instrument had to indicate that the scale was primarily designed to measure adaptive behavior. That is, tools such as the Developmental Profile II (Alpern, Boll, & Shearer, 1980), which was primarily designed for use as a screening tool for developmental deficits, were eliminated from consideration in this section. Second, at least one of the intended functions of the instrument had to involve usefulness for classification/placement decisions. This means, that at a minimum, norms were developed and cited, and at best, a stratified, representative national sample was used to generate norms for the comparison group. Third, the AB tool had to meet or attempt to meet most of the criteria set forth in the evaluation criteria discussed in the last section. AB instruments selected for review will be discussed in accordance with this five-step evaluative procedure.

Recovering the Wheel

There is an old adage that chastises the young for always trying to *reinvent the wheel* when all it really needed was some modification. The Adaptive Behavior Scale, School Edition (ABS-SE) (Lambert & Windmiller, 1981) represents heedance to that intergenerational caution. The ABS-SE represents revised procedures and expanded reference-group norms from the Adaptive Behavior Scale, Public School Version (Lambert, Windmiller, & Cole, 1975). Lambert and her colleagues recognized the need to develop an AB instrument that could aid in diagnosis, placement, and program planning for school-aged children. After reviewing AB instruments that were available in the early 1970s, it was decided that the AAMD ABS (Nihira et al., 1974) met most of the criteria except for its psychometric properties. Most of the content of the ABS was retained except for domestic activity and other minor changes.

Adaptive Behavior Scale, School Edition (ABS-SE)

Function. Diagnosis/screening, placement, instructional planning (an instructional planning grid is included), progress evaluation, Individualized Education Plan (IEP) development. The scale is designed for ages three through 16.

Content. The ABS-SE covers 22 skill areas and 11 domains of maladaptive behavior. The band of coverage is comprehensive.

Depth of coverage is fair. There is an adequate sample of nonschool behaviors.

Administrative method. The ABS-SE employs the indirect method with the teacher (preferred) or parent filling out the assessment booklet. The assessment booklet contains a general instruction section. Every item is filled out; there are no basal or ceiling rules. Training workshops are still occasionally available.

Psychometric characteristics. Norms were standardized on 6,500 persons between the ages of three and 16 from California and Florida. Reference group norms are available by chronological age and by school placement: Educable Mentally Retarded (EMR), Trainable Mentally Retarded (TMR), and regular. Summary results are expressed in three ways: percentile scores by domain, scaled scores across five factors, and cumulative percentages representing a comparison/composite adaptive behavior score. *Reliability/validity* are reported in a separate diagnostic and technical manual. Construct, content, and predictive validity studies are reported. Reliability coefficients are adequate. Standard error of measurements were computed on the factor scores by age and by three types of school placement (e.g., regular, EMR, TMR). The SEM's range from small to quite large. Therefore, the user should use caution in interpreting the factor scores.

Administrative considerations. Time of administration, according to the manual, is 15 to 45 minutes. The cost of the instrument and its accessories should be checked out with the publisher: Publishers Test Service, 2500 Garden Road, Monterey, CA 93940.

Strengths of the ABS-SE include its strong theoretical base, ample empirical research data available on the original instrument, the ABS, and standardization norms. One of the nicest features of the ABS-SE are factor scores which are computed and then graphed on a diagnostic profile sheet. The factor scores were derived from discriminant analyses on the raw scores. The five factor domains are: personal self-sufficiency, community self-sufficiency, personal-social responsibility, social adjustment, and personal adjustment. The administration and instruction planning manual to the ABS-SE contains a helpful resource guide to curriculum materials. There are two areas of weakness. First, there is no place on the factor profile to record the band of error or SEM; the SEM is not computed for scale or composite scores. Second, the depth of coverage for each domain is quite limited and, thus, it has limited utility for use in curriculum development.

Socioecological Approach

Mercer and her colleagues (Mercer, 1973; Lewis & Mercer, 1978; Mercer, 1979) emphasize that the development of the Adaptive Behavior Inventory for Children (ABIC) derives from a broad sociological framework. Further, she cautioned the potential user that results from the ABIC should only be interpreted within the larger context of her Multi-Cultural Pluralistic Assessment Model, which consists of nine separate measures. In brief, Mercer conceives of social adaptation as a dynamic process whereby the child behaviorally moves through a developmental sequence of six roles to meet the expectations of her reference group. Normal behavior is defined as role performance that meets these expectations. The ABIC is a method for obtaining a multidimensional, cross-sectional view of how well the child is performing each of these roles at a particular point in time compared to a culturally-relevant reference group. Role performance for the young child centers on the family, neighborhood and peer interaction. As the child gets into school, role performance embraces more nonschool roles. For the older child, community roles such as consumer/earner, social responsibility, and self-maintenance become central.

Adaptive Behavior Inventory for Children (ABIC)

Function. Primary function is identification/placement. The target population is children from the ages of five through 11 years.

Content. The band of coverage is comprehensive. Major skill areas are covered, but embedded in various role performances. Depth of coverage is moderately low; the author states that the ABIC is not intended to be used as a criterion-referenced measure. There are 242 items across six scales: family (e.g., helpful around the house, teaching younger siblings); community (e.g., move about the neighborhood); peer group (e.g., behavior and interaction with age peers that are nonfamily members); nonacademic school (e.g., behavior on the playground, interaction with classmates); earner/consumer (e.g., understanding money, shopping skills); and self-maintenance (e.g., impulse control, self-confidence, personal hygiene). The behavior specificity of the scale is rated as good.

Method of administration. The ABIC employs an indirect method, interview type. The scale is administered by a trained interviewer with the informant being the mother of the child, if possible. Training workshops are available. ABIC uses stringent standardized instructions and has basal and ceiling rules.

Psychometric characteristics. Norms were developed from a 2,085 standardization sample. The sample consisted of equal numbers of Hispanic, black, and white children. Thus, the sample should not be considered a stratified, representative sample of the U.S. population. Ethnic and socioeconomic differences on the ABIC are ambiguous. Norms were developed by age. *Reliability/validity* are reported, but are not always clear. Reliability coefficients and standard error of measurements for the six scaled scores are available by age and ethnic group. The SEM is not used in computing and displaying the scores on a profile sheet. Summary scores available are: scaled scores (which are difficult to interpret), percentile scores for the six subscales, and composite or total score which is derived by averaging the six scaled scores. A unique feature of the ABIC is a 24 item *veracity* subscale to check whether or not the informant is inflating the child's scores. There are also cutoff rules for validating the scale itself.

Administrative considerations. Time of administration for the ABIC is not reported in the manual. See the publisher for the cost of the instrument and its accompanying forms: The Psychological Corporation.

One of the advantages of the ABIC is its high ceiling. That is, it was particularly designed for differentiating children that perform adaptively in the mildly retarded range from children that are in the borderline range and above. However, by the same token, it would probably not be as useful in differentiating among the various levels of mental retardation. It was not intended nor should it be used as a basis for curriculum or program development.

Systems Approach

Three AB measurement systems are reviewed. They are grouped here because of the following common traits: (a) recent publication date, (b) product of rigorous, modern research techniques, (c) sophisticated technical and psychometric characteristics, (d) broad age range, and (e) attempt to assist the user through a broad continuum of function (i.e., screening tool, diagnosis, placement, program planning, program monitoring, program evaluation, etc.). Each of these scales will be reviewed separately.

The Scales of Independent Behavior (SIB)

Function. The SIB (Bruininks, Woodcock, Weatherman, & Hill, 1984) is intended to serve a comprehensive function. The target age range is from infant through adult.

Content. Band of coverage is comprehensive. The SIB consists of 226 items distributed among 14 subscales, four clusters (motor, social and communication skills, personal living skills, community living skills) which are combined to yield a measure of broad independence. In addition, there is a short form (32 items) for quick screening, an early development scale (32 items) for individuals whose developmental level is below 2-1/2 years, and a *problem behavior scale* (8 categories) which yields four maladaptive scores. Depth of coverage is increased because of the rigorous and systematic scoring scheme where each item is rated on a four point scale. Functional skills are covered at the upper ranges while developmental-type skills are covered at the lower ranges. Precise behavioral-referenced items make the SIB easier to rate than most other scales.

Method of administration. The SIB uses the indirect method, interview type. Detailed standardized instructions are employed with a easel-style test booklet. Basal and ceiling rules are included for each subdomain. Training workshops are available and highly recommended, particularly for scoring and interpretation.

Psychometric characteristics. Norms were derived from a standardized, stratified national sample of 1,670 individuals. Summary scores available include: percentile ranks, standard scores, age scores for the 14 subscales, instructional range, relative performance index (RPI), adjusted AB scores for cluster scales, full or composite scale, special scales, and four maladaptive index scores. *Reliability/validity* are reported in a separate technical manual. The manual cites extensive studies. The SEM is included in the profile summary.

Administrative considerations. The manual states that the total test takes approximately 45 to 60 minutes to administer. Each cluster or special scale takes from 10 to 15 minutes. For the cost of materials, see the publisher of the SIB: DLM, One DLM Park, Allen, TX 75002.

The SIB has a number of unique built-in features: (a) microcomputer scoring and profiling, (b) a flexible system of administration (each subscale can be administered separately), and (c) maladaptive behaviors are rated on two dimensions (severity, frequency) and are norm-referenced to a large handicapped population. The SIB is statistically and structurally linked to the Woodcock-Johnson Psycho-Educational Battery (1977). This allows the user to derive an adjusted individual adaptive behavior profile that considers age and cognitive ability simultaneously. One factor that needs further study is the SIB's ability to discriminate adaptive behavior performance between borderline and mildly mentally retarded adults. Webb (1985) has employed the SIB system as both an individual and program evaluation tool successfully in a work and socialization day program for adults with mental retardation.

The Vineland Adaptive Behavior Scale

The Vineland Adaptive Behavior Scale (VABS) (Sparrow, Balla, & Cicchetti, 1984a, 1984b) is another system that is intended for multipurpose user implementation. The title of the VABS suggests that it is a revision of the Vineland Social Maturity Scale, a scale that was discussed in a previous section of this chapter. However, there is very little commonality between the two scales. The one enduring aspect from Doll's VSMS (1953) is that data is gathered from the informant using a semistructured interview format.

Function. The authors identify three functions for the VSMS: diagnosis, program planning, and research. The target age range is from birth to 18 years-11 months and low functioning adults.

Content. The band of coverage is comprehensive. There are three versions of the VABS. The *Interview Edition, Survey Form* has 297 items. There are 11 skill subdomains grouped into four domains: communication, daily living skills, socialization, and motor skills. A maladaptive behavior domain contains 36 items. The *Interview Edition, Expanded Form* [italics added] consists of 577 items grouped in the same manner as the Survey Edition. A *Classroom Edition* consists of 244 items; its target age group is three through 12 years-11 months. The survey form is primarily designed for use as a diagnostic and screening tool, while the expanded version, because of its broader depth of coverage by skill area, can be useful in program planning, monitoring and evaluation. The authors employ a developmental framework for item selection. Overall, the items contain sufficient behavior-specificity which should allow for ease and reliability of scoring.

Method of administration. The VABS employs an indirect method, interview type. The VABS uses a semistructured interview method. Interviewers must be trained prior to administering the VABS. There are basal and ceiling rules for each version of the VABS. Training workshops are available and recommended. Scoring criteria are available in the manual.

Psychometric characteristics. Norms are standardized on a national stratified sample of 3,000 individuals from birth to 18 years-11 months. Norms were used both in developing the survey and expanded form. Norms for the Classroom Edition were computed from a representative sample of 3,000 children three years through 12 years-11 months. In addition, seven supplementary norms on special populations (e.g., mentally retarded adults, emotionally disturbed children) are also available on both the survey and expanded forms. Summary scores are reported by standard scores, percentile ranks, stanines, adaptive levels, and age equivalencies. Supplementary group norms are summarized by percentile ranks. *Reliability/ validity* are extensive and are reported in a separate technical manual. The standard error of measurement (SEM) is computed and represented in the profiles for the four major domains and for the composite score.

Administrative considerations. The survey form takes from 20 to 60 minutes to administer. The expanded form takes from 60 to 90 minutes. The Classroom Edition takes 20 minutes. For cost break-down of the VABS and its ancillary materials, consult the publisher: American Guidance Service, Circle Pines, MN 55014-1796.

In summary, the VABS is a broad measure of adaptive behavior that should prove useful for a number of functions. An instructional planning format, parent guide, and a microcomputer software package for scoring and profile display are additional features. As mentioned with some of the other instruments, its low ceiling makes the VABS a questionable measure for differentiating mildly handicapped from borderline or low average individuals. The user should be forewarned that the supplemental norms reported in the manual are based on a very small sample.

The Normative Adaptive Behavior Checklist (NABC) and the Comprehensive Test of Adaptive Behavior (CTAB)

The NABC and its companion the CTAB (Adams, 1984) are the final multipurpose AB assessment instruments reviewed in this section. This scale was first developed as a criterion referenced test, but was later expanded to encompass a broader use.

Function. The author states that the main purpose of the NABC is to assist the user in making placement decisions. Emphasis is placed on the development of an instrument that can be administered in a short amount of time. The CTAB was designed to be both a descriptive and prescriptive test useful in curriculum development for the handicapped population. The target age range for the NABC and CTAB is from birth to 21 years.

Content. The band of coverage is comprehensive. Both instruments assess six scale areas: self-help, home living, independent living, social, sensory and motor, language concepts, and academic skills. The NABC contains 120 items while the CTAB has a much higher depth of coverage in that it has 24 subcategories with approximately 500 items. Maladaptive behaviors are not included. Items are behavioral with accompanying specific criteria to help the interviewer give an accurate response.

Method of administration. The NABC employs an indirect method, third party type. The informant, typically a parent, fills out the questionnaire. If the informant is in doubt about a particular item, the author encourages direct testing of the skill in question. Responses are in a yes/no format. The CTAB has two forms, one for the teacher and another for the parent/guardian for the purpose of cross-checking. A record form allows the user to track the client's performance. Some of the language concepts and academic skills are tested directly.

Psychometric characteristics. For the NABC, *norms* are standardized on a national sample of 6,000 nonhandicapped individuals from birth to 21 years. For the CTAB, *norms* were computed from a national sample of 4,500 mentally retarded individuals from early childhood through old age. Summary scores are presented by standard scores, percentiles, and age equivalencies. *Reliability/validity* are reported in a separate technical manual. The standard error of measurements are reported in the technical manual by age and sex. They are not included in the profile.

Administrative considerations. The NABC can be administered in approximately 20 minutes. The CTAB administration time was not found in the manual. For cost information, see the publisher: Charles E. Merrill Publishing Co., 1300 Alum Creek Dr., Box 508, Columbus, OH 43216.

Adams outlines a step-by-step method to link scores on the CTAB to specific IEP objectives. The record form can be useful in tracking clients' progress. Machine scoring of the NABC is available.

Computerized Assessment and Management Systems Approach

The two scales reviewed in this section represent the application of microcomputer technology to AB measurement and program design. They are similar to other AB measurement system approaches in that they intend to serve a multi-use function. However, they differ in two important ways. First, while the SIB and VABS offer computer-assisted scoring and interpretation as a supplement for the user, these present scales are a component of a fully computerized system. Second, while both of the present scales allude to norm references, their emphasis is on using AB generated data, both individual and aggregate, to meet program and administrative needs.

The *California Adaptive Behavior Scale* (CABS) (Gardner & Breuer, 1984) is a component of a comprehensive, fully computerized data management system to guide clinical and administrative decision-making with developmentally disabled people.

Function. Its aim is comprehensive. CABS has limited usefulness for diagnostic/placement decisions. The target age range is all ages.

Content. The band of coverage is representative. The full scale consists of 329 items divided into 24 adaptive behavior skill domains. Depth of coverage is below average. Three clinical scales are derived from the full scale: (a) adaptive age scale consisting of 144 items, (b) school readiness scale consisting of 90 items, and (c) work readiness scale consisting of 105 items. Maladaptive behaviors are surveyed by a separate assessment component.

Method of administration. The CABS uses the indirect method, third party type. Scoring guidelines are provided. The informant selects the highest level of performance in each of 24 areas. No training is necessary to complete the scale. The scale can be computer administered and scored.

Psychometric characteristics. No independent *norms* are cited in the manual. Items are assigned age equivalencies. Summary scores in the form of age equivalencies are available for each domain. Profiles (the highest level of achievement) across domains present an individual's strengths and weaknesses. A unique feature of the CABS is that it has two internal validity scales that can be computed for each test administration: internal reliability score and internal validity score. *Reliability/validity* are cited but based on a small sample.

Administrative considerations. According to the manual, the time of administration is 15 minutes. For cost breakdown, see the publisher: Planet Press, P.O. Box 3477, Newport Beach, CA 92663-3418.

The CABS and its other components are in the process of evolving. This adaptive behavior system appears most useful for individual program planning and tracking purposes. Another unique feature is the availability of computer software to generate reports (e.g., psychological, individual program plan).

The *Fairview Adaptive Behavior Scale* (FABS) (Foster & Barron, 1985a) is a component of an assessment, training, and management microcomputer system called the Fairview Adaptive Individualized Record (FAIR) (Foster & Barron, 1985b), for use with developmentally disabled persons. Since the FAIR is not commercially available yet, a narrative summary of the tool will be presented. The FAIR consists of 1,274 behavior-specific items across eight domains: self-care, socialization, communication, leisure, sensorimotor, vocational, academic, and independent living. The FABS is a 108-item subtest of the larger scale which serves as an initial screening tool. The FABS is completed by a third party. The FAIR employs a branching approach in displaying strengths and deficits. This gives the user access to more fine-tuned scale items to permit more precise location of deficits. Items are norm-referenced by age equivalencies. The source for norm-referencing, as well as reliability and validity data, is not cited in materials available for review. Item selection was based on both developmental and functional models. Unique features of the FABS include: a relative average difficulty index for each item that allows the user to select from training objectives that have comparable levels of difficulty, a report generation feature that can link the FAIR to other scales (e.g., the ABS, Camelot). Adapted versions of the scale are designed for use with other kinds of handicaps (e.g., visual, orthopedic, etc.).

Direct Assessment Approach

There has been a history of disagreement among researchers in the field of AB measurement on the best method to obtain reliable data about an individual's adaptive level (Walls et al., 1977; Spreat et al., 1983). Most scales either employ the interview or third party method of data collection. Balthazar (1971) has been a strong advocate for direct observational methods. Indirect methods have been criticized for their dependence on the perception and/or memory of the informant, observer bias, and lack of scale item specificity (Linkenhoker & McCarron, 1980). However, direct observation can be time consuming and may only allow a narrow band of domain coverage.

In response to these concerns, AB measurement tools such as the Social and Prevocational Information Battery (SPIB) (Halpern,

Raffeld, Irvin, & Link, 1975); Test of Social Inference (TSI) (Edmonson, deJung, Leland, & Leach, 1974); Childrens Adaptive Behavior Scale (CABS) (Kicklighter, Bailey, & Richmond, 1980); and the Street Survival Skills Questionnaire (SSSQ) (Linkenhoker & McCarron, 1980) have been developed to gather adaptive behavior data more directly. For example, on the CABS, a child is required to give verbal responses to a series of questions concerning five areas: language development, independent functioning, family role performance, economics, and socialization. The SSSQ will be reviewed as representative of this trend in AB measurement. The authors point out that the SSSQ was not intended to be a comprehensive measurement of adaptive behavior, but to focus on more community relevant functional skills. The SSSQ is part of the McCarron-Dial Work Evaluation System (McCarron & Dial, 1976).

Street Survival Skills Questionnaire (SSSQ)

Function. Classification, diagnosis, placement, and program planning are identified in the manual as primary functions of this tool. The target age range is from 9 years-6 months to 40 years.

Content. The band and depth of coverage is limited to functional community skills. However, when the SSSQ is used in conjunction with the McCarron-Dial system, its band of coverage increases considerably. The scale itself consists of 216 items, grouped conceptually into 29 subdomains which collapses into nine subscales: basic concepts, functional signs, tools, domestic management, health/first aid/safety, public services, time, money, and measurements. Items within each subscale are ordered from easy to hard.

Method of administration. The SSSQ employs the direct method. It uses standardized testing procedures. Each question is read aloud. The informant points to one of four possible answers. There are no basal and ceiling rules.

Psychometric characteristics. Two sets of *norms* were developed: normal children and adults (9 years-6 months through 40 years); and mentally retarded individuals (15 years to 55 years). Norms were based on small samples. Individual test results need to be interpreted, therefore, with caution. Scaled scores are available for each of the nine subscales. A survival skills quotient ($x = 100$,

SQ = 15) represents a composite score which can be displayed in a graph form. *Reliability/validity* studies are cited only for the neuropsychologically disabled. The SEMs are computed for each subscale and the total score, but are not used in the profiles.

Administrative considerations. Time of administration is between 45 minutes and one hour. For costs, see the publisher: Common Market Press, P.O. Box 45628, Dallas, TX 75245.

The SSSQ is a nonverbal, direct measure of some functional components of adaptive behavior. Used in conjunction with the McCarron-Dial system it is useful in residential and vocational placement decisions for developmentally disabled adults. A master planning chart provides a pictorial display of strengths and deficits to aid in individual program planning. While most other adaptive behavior scales measure performance (i.e., what a person does), the SSSQ evaluates adaptive knowledge (i.e., what a person is capable of doing).

Specialized Population Approach

The AB measurement tools presented in this section have been in existence for some time. All report some type of reference group norms, typically derived from a sample of mentally retarded. These instruments have endured because professionals in the field have found them useful in clinical settings despite psychometric limitations and norm-referencing inadequacies. It is the issue, not the psychometric sophistication of the instrument, that should guide AB tool selection. Not all issues dealing with identification/placement require comparisons of individual performance to national norms. For example, a clinician may be interested in determining which of three alternative residential training programs to place a client. In this case, an AB scale that is norm-referenced to mentally retarded children or adults may be the most useful comparison to determine entry into the appropriate program.

For individuals who are classified as severely to profoundly mentally retarded, much of the training has been directed towards the acquisition of basic skills (e.g., dressing, toileting) that normal children of three to five years of age are expected to master. Since most AB measures attempt to cover a broad developmental range, typically from birth to 18 years of age, they are of little help in developing program objectives for the severe to profound mentally retarded. The following AB instruments are designed to assess severe to profound performance deficits and have produced reference-norms appropriate to this group: Fairview Self-Help Scale (Ross, 1969); Balthazar Scales of Adaptive Behavior (BSAB) (Balthazar, 1973); the TARC Assessment Inventory for Severely Handicapped Children (Sailor & Mix, 1975); Progress Assessment Chart (P-A-C) (Gunzburg, 1976); and Wisconsin Behavior Rating Scale (WBRS) (Song & Jones, 1979). While the band of content coverage for most of these scales is comprehensive, it is their depth of coverage that gives them a clear advantage in program planning, monitoring and evaluating individuals with severe to profound mental retardation and/or severe handicaps. The BSAB and WBRS endorse a direct type of observation, while the others employ both direct and indirect methods.

The Cain-Levine Social Competency Scale (Cain, Levine, & Elzey, 1963) employs an indirect method, interview type to gather adaptive behavior data on moderately retarded children between the ages of five and 13 years of age.

The AAMD ABS (Nihira et al., 1974); P-A-C 1A, P-A-C 2 (Gunzburg, 1976); and the Camelot Behavioral Checklist (CBC) (Foster, 1977) are useful for individuals with milder handicaps (e.g., mild mental retardation). The CBC consists of 399 items grouped into 40 subdomains and 10 summary domains, similar to the ABS Part I domains. Band and depth of coverage are adequate. The indirect method, third party type, is the primary method of data collection. The use of direct probes is suggested where uncertainty exists. Norm-references are not clearly presented in the manual, but presumably are based on a sample of institutionalized mentally retarded. Reliability and validity data are cited. Two features of the CBC aid in its usefulness for program planning. First, a difficulty of training index based on the percentage of individuals in the sample that required training on a particular scale item was developed. This index can be used to assist the user in identifying skill objective priorities. Second, a skill acquisition program bibliography (Foster, Lewis, Tucker, Foster, & Gentry, 1979) links each item on the CBC with commercially available training/intervention curriculum.

CURRENT ISSUES IN ADAPTIVE BEHAVIOR
MEASUREMENT

Moos (1974) writing prophetically about the impending burst of clinical and research activity that would take place within the 1970s and 1980s in the measurement of adaptive behavior stated, "the exponential growth of the area over the last several years makes it a relatively safe prediction that it will skip the latency stage and will soon blossom into a full growth adolescent identity crisis" (p. 335). This identity crisis is in full blossom now. Legislation, litigation, and the current political climate combine to pressure the field of adaptive behavior to live up to its *presumed* usefulness. Establishing credibility and viability are rapidly becoming important issues, particularly in the light of recent criticism from Zigler, Balla, & Hodapp (1984) who advocate for the removal of adaptive behavior from the classification scheme of mental retardation.

The usefulness of AB instruments in classifying (e.g., normal vs. mentally retarded) and placing (e.g., regular classes vs. special education) individuals, exemplifies the magnitude of problems faced in the adaptive behavior field's *adolescence.* For example, consider the issue of prevalence rates of mental retardation in the general population. There is a current consensus among major classification manuals that *concurrent* deficits in intelligence and adaptive behavior must be present in order to diagnose mental retardation. Mercer (1973) found that sole reliance on IQ measures led to an over representation of blacks and Hispanics who were classified as mentally retarded and placed in special education classes. She found that imposition of this two-dimensional (i.e., IQ + adaptive behavior) definition led to significantly reduced and more ethnically balanced estimates of the prevalence of mental retardation. Adaptive behavior measures have been touted as the cornerstone, therefore, of nonbiased assessment.

Yet placing measures of adaptive behavior on a diagnostic parity with older, more established methods of evaluation such as the IQ has its problems. There still remains wide disagreement around fundamental adaptive behavior issues such as definition, administrative procedures, standardization, reliability, and validity (Coulter & Morrow, 1978). Zigler et al. (1984) point out that disagreements over the definition of adaptive behavior produce national prevalence rates of mental retardation that can range from 100,000 to 4 million. This wide disparity makes the two-dimensional classification scheme seem almost useless for developing nationwide resources and conducting long-range planning for persons with mental retardation. In this section, some conceptual and methodological issues that could either impede progress or enhance the growth of the AB measurement field will be discussed.

Conceptual Considerations

Probably one of the most lingering controversies among practitioners and researchers in developmental disabilities centers around the usefulness of measuring adaptive behavior. The controversy heats up when the issue involves classification/placement, but cools down somewhat when the issue is program planning/intervention. How do IQ and adaptive behavior differ? What is the relationship between adaptive behavior and IQ? Does information generated from AB measurement instruments describe something significant about the individual that was not already known or that could have been predicted from other preexisting measures? Spreat et al. (1983) present empirical research on both sides of this complex issue. Grossman (1983) outlines two conceptual differences between IQ and AB measures. He states that IQ tests attempt to determine the highest potential for performance by emphasizing language, reasoning, and abstract abilities. On the other hand, AB instruments attempt to determine common and routine performance by emphasizing basic, daily living skills such as eating, dressing, and toileting. Some researchers argue that adaptive behavior becomes a more critical and independent dimension with mentally retarded living in the community (Leland, 1978), with individuals who have an IQ above 50 (Meyers et al., 1979), and with ethnic minorities (Mercer, 1973). However, others assert that AB measurement is a redundant, conceptually vague, time consuming, psychometrically primitive measure of general intelligence (Baumeister & Muma, 1975; Zigler et al., 1984). Zigler et al. (1984) have recently argued for the abandonment of AB measurement in the classification scheme of mental retardation in favor of the IQ. In fact, despite the inclusion of adaptive behavior in the AAMD Classification Manual since 1959, they report that researchers and practitioners still rely primarily on the IQ for classification purposes.

Concurrent with the struggle to secure adaptive behavior its own unique identity within the broader field of diagnostic classification of individuals, is a model that presupposes the validity of the adaptive behavior concept. This model advocates combining AB measurement with IQ and other measures through statistical linkages in order to increase predictive and generalization power. For example, the Woodcock-Johnson Psycho-Educational Battery Part Four (Bruininks et al., 1984) covaried cognitive ability, age, and adaptive behavior in order to obtain an adjusted adaptive behavior index score for individuals. This approach holds promise, yet it does not go far enough. Although most contemporary AB scales include a measure of maladaptive behavior, separate scores are typically reported for this domain. Yet, in real life, an individual's level of perceived social competence is determined by both skill performance and behavior adjustment. A nine-year-old child that manifests academic proficiency in one setting, but lacks temper control across settings, will rarely be seen as competent. Linkenhoker and McCarron (1980) attempted to consider social knowledge, skill performance and behavior maladjustment simultaneously. He and his colleagues developed a multiple regression formula to predict residential placement needs of handicapped adults. Much more empirical research is needed in this multidimensional approach to assessment.

Most conceptual and empirical research in AB measurement has been concerned with separating retarded from normal performance and in establishing levels of retarded adaptive performance. There has been little concern in differentiating mild, borderline, and low average adaptive deficits. This takes on added importance when human service agencies have to make tough decisions among these catagories in order to establish or deny services to individuals. For example, California Regional Centers mandated by the state to provide advocacy and program coordination services to the developmentally disabled, must deny assistance to individuals in the borderline range of adaptive behavior. Yet, what distinguishes the borderline from the mild performer on adaptive behavior remains unclear. The problem is that AB scales are generally negatively skewed. This means that there are more items at the lower levels of performance, and there are fewer items at the higher levels of performance. This produces less discrimination power at these higher levels. Except for anthropological studies such as Edgerton's (1967) *Cloak of Competence*, very little is known about the area of adaptive functioning that lies between normal and retarded performance.

Negative skewing of AB scales also has an effect on the program planning/intervention usefulness of these measurement tools as applied to higher functioning individuals. That is, most AB instruments tend to emphasize basic, core living skills. Inclusion of these skills is an attractive psychometric feature because they are easily identifiable, observable, and quantifiable. At present, items focusing on self-concept, motivation, and social awareness are often missing or covered superficially. These are often the variables that are most likely essential for discriminating between mild, borderline and low average levels of social competence. The use of these scales to generate program planning activities for people with mild handicaps is limited. For example, training objectives that are derived from the socialization domain of most AB measures neglect social interfacing skills (i.e., social conversation, assertiveness, social manners) that are highly desirable for community integration.

Measures of adaptive behavior have exclusively relied on a cross-sectional approach. That is, social adaptation is estimated by assessing an individual's functioning at a specific point in time. Age and, sometimes, sex and other demographic variables may be considered. However, this is less than ideal. Social competency has to do with temporal continuity as well. Lewis and Mercer (1978) point out that optimal measures of adaptive behavior would involve the development of a longitudinal chart which tracks the child's movement through the various social systems. This type of data collection would be extremely helpful in validating the utility of the cross-sectional approach which is in such common use today. Repeating AB measures at various times in an individual's development is a starting point, but falls short.

The adaptive level of the *individual* has been the focal point upon which adaptive behavior has been conceptualized and measured.

Classification schemes and program planning are also built around the functional autonomy of the individual. Yet, it is commonly accepted that families, for example, can capture the complementary strengths of individual members while compensating for the deficits of individual members. That is, the family or group may project a more socially competent image than any individual member. Cohen and Leland (1977) studied a number of severely handicapped, institutionalized men who had bonded together to form a *Workshop Group*. Evaluated individually on a adaptive behavior measure, 77% of the men were classified in the severe range of adaptive functioning. Yet, when evaluated as a group, only mild deficits were noted. Using this broader perspective, program planning for the group might concentrate on increasing democratic decision-making processes (i.e., fair and representative decisions). Implications from such a study can be far reaching and provocative. Evaluating the adaptive behavior status of groups and couples may provide insights to new training approaches toward fostering interdependent living.

Methodological Considerations

The young field of AB measurement has had to constantly fend off criticism regarding its lack of technical rigor in scale development. Recently published and well researched AB scales such as the SIB (Bruininks et al., 1984) and the VABS (Sparrow et al., 1984a) have made significant strides toward meeting some of these historical objections. Methodological questions still remain which, if not addressed satisfactorily, will block the field's ability to endure as a viable, useful measure of human performance. Three of these methodological tangles will be discussed in this section: multiple raters vs. single rater, third part vs. direct assessment, and reliance on single scores vs. multiple scores.

As the reader will recall, inter-rater reliability is one of the most standard statistics used to establish a scale's usefulness. Most of the AB scales cited in this chapter report inter-rater reliability coefficients and most are considered adequate, ranging from the .80s to .90s. However, as Spreat et al. (1983) point out, the average inter-rater reliability of a specific item in a scale may be considerably lower. This should significantly reduce the confidence of the user when the intent of AB measurement is toward goal planning and training. Secondly, colleagues of the author have complained regularly that reliance on one informant (rater) places unrealistic expectations on that person's observation skills and her experience with the client across environments (e.g., classroom, home, etc.). This becomes a particular problem when the teacher is asked to rate the child on nonschool domains. The use of two or more raters or even group ratings could significantly increase the confidence in the quality of the measurement (Spreat et al., 1983).

Even with the utilization of multiple raters and rigorous reliability research on the more recent AB measurement instruments, some psychologists still feel uncomfortable relying on third party or interview data to make judgments about a person's adaptive behavior level. They would prefer a more direct approach such as the administration of a test or the opportunity of observing the individual. To dispel some doubts about sole reliance on indirect methods of data collection, the author proposes two clinical strategies. First, when feasible, some or all scales of the SSSQ, a more direct measure, may be combined with a third party assessment such as the VABS or SIB. Second, after the standard administration of an AB indirect measurement is completed, the rater can choose to conduct direct probes of the client by randomly selecting items from the scale. This yields a reliability check between the informant and an individual's actual performance on the selected items. One of the most promising approaches is that taken by Gardner and Breuer (1984). The CABS builds in an internal reliability and validity scale much like clinicians are accustomed to doing on standard clinical instruments such as the Minnesota Multiphasic Personality Inventory (MMPI) (Hathaway & McKinley, 1967). This whole area needs more research and clinical attention.

A final methodological concern centers on the usefulness of adaptive behavior overall scores versus domain scores. While the former are perceived as having utility primarily in classification and identification, the latter is perceived as useful in program planning and intervention. Most of the newer scales allow the user to perform both functions with the same instrument. But the question still remains whether or not a single score can truly represent such a diverse set of behaviors ranging from being able to dress independently to being able to answer an ad for a job. Spreat et al. (1983) present a discussion of this controversy in their chapter on AB measurement. One approach that may be worth investigating is that of a profile analysis used by MMPI and other clinical tools. That is, rather than relying on a single score, scores across domains are examined for patterns that fit certain diagnostic criteria. The ABS-SE factor scores (Lambert & Windmiller, 1981) are an initial attempt in that direction.

REFERENCES

Adams, G. L. (1984). *Technical Manual: CTAB, NABC*. Columbus: Charles E. Merrill Publishing Co.

Alpern, G. D., Boll, Thomas J., & Shearer, M. S. (1980). *Developmental Profile II Manual*. Aspen, CO: Psychological Development Publications.

American Psychiatric Association (1980). *Diagnostic and Statistical Manual of Mental Disorders DSM = III* (3rd Edition). Washington, DC: American Psychiatric Association.

Balthazar, E. E. (1971). The assessment of adaptive behavior. In D. A. Primrose (Ed.), *Proceedings of the Second Congress of the International Association for the Scientific Study of Mental Deficiency*. Surrey, England: Michael Jackson.

Balthazar, E. E. (1973). *Balthazar Scales of Adaptive Behavior*. Palo Alto, CA: Consulting Psychologists Press.

Baumeister, A. A., & Muma, J. R. (1975). On defining mental retardation. *Journal of Special Education*, 9, 293-306.

Blatt, B., & Kaplan, F. (1966). *Christmas in purgatory: A photographic essay on mental retardation*. Boston: Allyn & Bacon.

Boone, R. (1983). Legislation and litigation. In R. E. Schmid & L. M. Magata (Eds.), *Contemporary issues in special education* (pp. 40-58). New York: Mc-Graw-Hill Associates.

Bruininks, R. H., Thurlow, M. L., Thurman, S. K., & Fiorelli, J. S. (1980). Deinstitutionalization and community services. In J. Wortis (Ed.), *Mental retardation and developmental disabilities* (Vol. XI) (pp. 55-101). New York: Brunner/Mazel.

Bruininks, R. H., Woodcock, R. W., Weatherman, R. F., & Hill, B. K. (1984). *Scales of Independent Behavior: Woodcock-Johnson Psycho-Educational Battery Part Four*. Allen, TX: DLM Training Resources.

Butterfield, E. (1976). Some basic changes in residential facilities. In R. B. Kugel, & A. Shearer (Eds.), *Changing patterns in residential services for the mentally retarded* (pp. 15-34). Washington, DC: President's Committee on Mental Retardation.

Cain, L. F., Levine, S., & Elzey, F. F. (1963). *Manual for the Cain-Levin Social Competency Scale*. Palo Alto, CA: Consulting Psychologists Press.

Cohen, H. G., & Leland, H. (1977). The workshop group: A case history of group processes among institutionalized mentally retarded men. *Mental Retardation, 15*, 45-46.

Coulter, W. A., & Morrow, H. W. (1978a). A collection of adaptive behavior measures. In W. A. Coulter, & H. S. Morrow (Eds.), *Adaptive behavior: Concepts and measurements* (pp. 141-156). New York: Grune & Stratton.

Coulter, W. A., & Morrow, H. W. (Eds.) (1978b). *Adaptive behavior: Concepts and measurements*. New York: Grune & Stratton.

Dingman, H. F. (1973). Foreword in J. R. Mercer, *Labeling the mentally retarded*. Berkeley: University of California Press.

Doll, E. A. (1953). *Measurement of social competence*. Circle Pines, MN: American Guidance Services, Inc.

Edgerton, R. B. (1967). *The cloak of competence: Stigma in the lives of the mentally retarded*. Berkeley: University of California Press.

Edmonson, B., deJung, J., Leland, H., & Leach, E. M. (1974). *The test of social inference*. Baldwin, NY: Educational Activities, Inc.

Foster, C., & Barron, J. (1985a). *Fairview Adaptive Behavior Scale*. Costa Mesa, CA: Fairview Developmental Community.

Foster, C., & Barron, J. (1985b). *Fairview Adaptive Individualized Record*. Costa Mesa, CA: Fairview Developmental Community.

Foster, C. D., Lewis, P. J., Tucker, D. J., Foster, R. W., & Gentry, B. (1979). *Skill acquisition program bibliography* (2nd Edition). Bellevue, WA: Edmark Associates.

Foster, R. (1977). *Camelot Behavioral Checklist Manual*. Bellevue, WA: Edmark Associates.

Gardner, J. M., & Breuer, A. M. (1984). *California Adaptive Behavior Scale Manual*. Newport Beach, CA: Planet Press Enterprises.

Gesell, A., & Amatruda, C. S. (1941). *Developmental diagnosis: Normal and abnormal child development*. New York: Hoeber.

Grossman, H. J. (Ed.) (1973). *Manual on Terminology and Classification in Mental Retardation* (Special Publication No. 2). Washington, DC: American Association on Mental Deficiency.

Grossman, H. J. (Ed.) (1983). *Classification in mental retardation*. Washington, DC: American Association on Mental Deficiency.

Gunzburg, H. C. (1973). *Social competence and mental handicap, an introduction to social education*. Baltimore: Williams & Wilkins.

Gunzburg, H. C. (1976). *Progress Assessment Chart of Social and Personal Development Manual* (4th Edition). Warwickshire, England: Sefa Ltd.

Halpern, A., Raffeld, P., Irvin, L., & Link, R. (1975). *Examiner's Manual for the Social and Prevocational Information Battery*. Monterey, CA: McGraw-Hill.

Hathaway, S. R., & McKinley, J. C. (1967). *The Minnesota Multiphasic Personality Inventory* (Rev. Manual). New York: Psychological Corporation.

Heber, R. A. (1959). A Manual on Terminology and Classification in Mental Retardation. *American Journal of Mental Deficiency*, 64. Monograph Supplement.

Heber, R. (1961). Modifications in the Manual on Terminology and Classification in Mental Retardation. *American Journal of Mental Deficiency* 65, 499-500.

International classification of diseases, 9th revision, clinical modification (1980). Washington, DC: U.S. Government Printing Office.

Kicklighter, R. H., Bailey, B. S., & Richmond, B. O. (1980). A direct measure of adaptive behavior. *School Psychology Review*, 9, 168-173.

Kugel, R. B., & Wolfensberger, W. (Eds.) (1969). *Changing patterns in residential services for the mentally retarded*. Washington, DC: President's Committee on Mental Retardation.

Kugel, R. B., & Shearer, A. (Eds.) (1976). *Changing patterns in residential services for the mentally retarded* (Rev.). Washington, DC: President's Committee on Mental Retardation.

Lambert, N. M., & Windmiller, M. (1981). *AAMD Adaptive Behavior Scale, School Edition*. Washington, DC: American Association on Mental Deficiency.

Lambert, N. M., Windmiller, M., & Cole, L. J. (1975). *AAMD Adaptive Behavior Scale, Public School Version*. Washington, DC: American Association on Mental Deficiency.

Leland, H. (1972). Mental retardation and adaptive behavior. *Journal of Special Education*, 6, 71-80.

Leland, H. (1973). Adaptive behavior and mentally retarded behavior. In C. E. Meyers, R. K. Eyman, & G. Tarjan (Eds.), *Socio-behavioral studies in mental retardation: Papers in honor of Harvy F. Dingman*. Washington, DC: American Association on Mental Deficiency.

Leland, H. (1978). Theoretical considerations of adaptive behavior. In W. A. Coulter, & H. W. Morrow (Eds.), *Adaptive behavior: Concepts and measurements* (pp. 21-44). New York: Grune & Stratton.

Lewis, J. F., & Mercer, J. R. (1978). The System of Multi-Cultural Pluralistic Assessment: SOMPA. In W. A. Coulter, & H. W. Morrow (Eds.), *Adaptive behavior: Concepts and measurements* (pp. 185-212). New York: Grune & Stratton.

Linkenhoker, D., & McCarron, L. (1980). *Adaptive Behavior: The Street Survival Skills Questionnaire*. Dallas, TX: Common Market Press.

Martin, R. (1979). *Educating handicapped children: The legal mandate*. Champaign, IL: Research Press.

Mayeda, T., Pelzer, I., & Van Zuylen, J. E. (1978). *Performance measures of skill and adaptive competencies in the developmentally disabled*. Pomona, CA: UCLA: The Neuropsychiatric Institute Research Group at Pacific State Hospital.

McCarron, L., & Dial, J. (1976). *McCarron-Dial Work Evaluation System*. Dallas: Common Market Press.

Mercer, J. R. (1973). *Labeling the mentally retarded: clinical and social system perspectives on mental retardation.* Berkeley: University of California Press.

Mercer, J. R. (1975). Sociocultural factors in educational labeling. In M. J. Begab, & S. A. Richardson (Eds.), *The mentally retarded and society: A social science perspective.* Baltimore: University Park Press.

Mercer, J. R. (1978). Theoretical constructs of adaptive behavior: Movement from a medical to a social-ecological perspective. In W. A. Coulter & H. W. Morrow (Eds.), *Adaptive behavior: Concepts and measurements* (pp. 59-82). New York: Grune & Stratton.

Mercer, J. R. (1979). *SOMPA Technical Manual.* New York: The Psychological Corporation.

Meyers, C. W., Nihira, K., & Zetlin, A. (1979). The measurement of adaptive behavior. In N. Ellis (Ed), *Handbook of mental deficiency, psychological theory and research* (2nd Edition). Hillsdale, NJ: Lawrence Erlbaum Associates.

Moos, R. H. (1974). Psychological techniques in assessment of adaptive behavior. In G. V. Coelho, D. A. Hamburg, & J. E. Adams (Eds.), *Coping and adaptation* (pp. 334-399). New York: Basic Books.

Morrow, H. W., & Coulter, W. A. (1978). A practitioner's approach to selecting adaptive behavior scales. In W. A. Coulter, & H. W. Morrow (Eds.), *Adaptive behavior: Concepts and measurements* (pp. 115-140). New York: Grune & Stratton.

Nihira, K., Foster, R., Shellhaas, M., & Leland, H. (1974). *American Association on Mental Deficiency Adaptive Behavior Scale.* Washington, DC: American Association on Mental Deficiency.

Nihira, K. (1978). Factorial descriptions of the AAMD Adaptive Behavior Scale. In W. A. Coulter, & H. W. Morrow (Eds.), *Adaptive behavior: Concepts and measurements* (pp 45-58). New York: Grune & Stratton.

Nirje, B. (1976). The normalization principle. In R. B. Kugel, & A. Shearer (Eds.), *Changing patterns in residential services for the mentally retarded* (pp 231-240). Washington, DC: President's Committee on Mental Retardation.

Piaget, J. (1952). *The origins of intelligence in children.* New York: International Universities Press.

President's Committee on Mental Retardation (1976). *The six-hour retarded child.* Washington, DC: U.S. Government Printing Office.

Ross, R. T. (1969). *Fairview Self-Help Scale.* Costa Mesa, CA: Fairview State Hospital.

Sailor, W., & Mix, B. (1975). *TARC Assessment System.* Lawrence, KS: H&H Enterprises.

Sarason, S. B., & Doris, J. (1969). *Psychological problems in mental deficiency* (4th Edition). New York: Harper & Row.

Song, A. Y., & Jones, S. (1979). *Wisconsin Behavior Rating Scale.* Madison, WI: Central Wisconsin Center for the Developmentally Disabled.

Song, A. Y., & Jones, S. E. (1982). Vineland Social Maturity Scale examined: The Wisconsin experience with 0-to-3 year old children. *American Journal of Mental Deficiency,* 86, 428-431.

Sparrow, S. S., Balla, D. A., & Cicchetti, D. V. (1984a). *Vineland Adaptive Scales, Interview Edition, Expanded Form Manual.* Circle Pines, MN: American Guidance Service.

Sparrow, S. S., Balla, D. A., & Cicchetti, D. V. (1984b). *Vineland Adaptive Behavior Scales, Interview Edition, Survey Form Manual.* Circle Pines, MN: American Guidance Service.

Spreat, S., Roszkowski, M. J., & Isett, R. D. (1983). Assessment of adaptive behavior in the mentally retarded. In S. E. Breuning, J. L. Matson, & R. P. Barrett (Eds.), *Advances in mental retardation and developmental disabilities* (Vol. 1). Greenwich, CT: JAI Press, Inc.

Standards for educational and psychological testing (1985). Washington, DC: American Psychological Association.

Terman, L. M. (1916). *The assessment of intelligence.* Boston: Houghton Mifflin.

Turnbull, H. P., & Turnbull, A. P. (1979). *Free appropriate public education law and implementation.* Denver: Love Publishing Co.

Walls, R. T., Werner, R. J., Bacon, A., & Zane, G. (1977). Behavior Checklists. In J. D. Cone, & R. P. Hawkins (Eds.), *Behavioral assessment: New directions in clinical psychology.* New York: Brunner/Mazel.

Webb, J. (1985). Personal communication.

Wolfensberger, W. (1969). The origin and nature of our institutional models. In R. B. Kugel, & W. Wolfensberger (Eds.), *Changing patterns in residential services for the mentally retarded.* Washington, DC: President's Committee on Mental Retardation.

Wolfensberger, W. (1976). The origin and nature of our institutional models. In R. B. Kugel, & A. Shearer (Eds.), *Changing patterns in residential services for the mentally retarded* (pp 35-82). Washington, DC: President's Committee on Mental Retardation.

Woodcock, R. W., & Johnson, M. B. (1977). *Woodcock-Johnson Psycho-Educational Battery.* Allen, TX: Teaching Resources.

Zigler, E., Balla, D., & Hodapp, R. (1984). On the definition and classification of mental retardation. *American Journal of Mental Deficiency*, 89, 215-230.

Functional Skills and Behavioral Technology: Identifying What to Train and How to Train It

Ennio Cipani

ABSTRACT. The present paper provides a technology for addressing two important questions in teaching/training exceptional individuals: (a) What to teach? and (b) How to teach it? A functional skills approach to identifying target skills is presented and contrasted with a developmental approach to training curriculum. A behavioral approach to training is delineated, in particular shaping and chaining methods for developing new behaviors. The use of these methodologies in working with handicapped individuals will lead to these people transitioning more successfully into the mainstream of society.

Allowing handicapped people to interact with the mainstream of society to their fullest extent is a civil right. How to effect this is the responsibility of public and private agencies who serve the handicapped. Personnel who teach and train handicapped children and youth to live in their least restrictive environment need to consider two factors: (a) what to teach (e.g., target skills) and (b) how to teach (i.e., the target skills). The field of education and training has gone through many phases and ideologies with respect to treatment and education of handicapped people. This chapter provides separate sections which address each of these issues with current knowledge and principles.

Ennio Cipani is affiliated with the Department of Special Education, University of the Pacific, Stockton, CA 95211.

TEACHING FUNCTIONAL SKILLS: WHAT TO TEACH

The current emphasis in designing habilitative and teaching environments for handicapped people is to teach/train skills that are required by their current and future environments. The term *functional skills* is used to refer to skills that allow handicapped people to more successfully interact in their natural environments (Brown, Branston, Baumgart, Vincent, Falvey, & Schroeder, 1979). These skills, once developed, increase the individual's capability and independence in his/her environment. The teaching environment should identify which skills are most needed by the handicapped person to sustain or increase effective social interaction with the environment. Previous habilitation models believed that individuals demonstrating delayed functioning must "pass through" prerequisite stages of intellectual development prior to being able to acquire functional, age-appropriate behaviors. The present functional skills model utilizes a "top-down" analysis (Snell, 1983) in identifying skills that need to be trained. In this manner, habilitative and educational plans will seek to teach skills which will lead more quickly to interaction (to some extent) with nonhandicapped peers in age-appropriate activities.

What Is a Top-Down Analysis?

A top-down analysis should produce training and curriculum programs that are age-appropriate, i.e., the skills being trained are selected as a function of the age of the child or youth. For example, a five-year-old child who is functioning at the profound level of retardation would require an habilitative and training environment that is considerably different than that of an 18-year-old profoundly retarded individual. Yet, until recently, habilitative efforts would group these individuals as homogenous in terms of programming needs.

In identifying an individual's deficits, four domains are analyzed as to their behavioral requirements: (a) vocational, (b) leisure/recreational, (c) domestic, and (d) community. These four domains are further subdivided: (a) natural environments within each domain, (b) subenvironments within each natural environment, (c) activities within each subenvironment, and (d) skills within each activity.

The use of this "top-down" analysis of deficit skills is presented below, using a hypothetical 18-year-old mildly retarded male as a case for illustration purposes.

Within the domestic domain, the natural environment would be his main residence. In this hypothetical case, it is a community group home, where he lives with five other developmentally disabled adolescents. Other domestic environments might include the residences of his natural parents or other relatives (if he spends time there periodically). For purposes of brevity, only the group home will be used in this case.

The analysis of subenvironments of this natural environment might reveal the following: the kitchen, dining room, laundry area, living room, bedroom, etc. The next step is to analyze activities that occur within each subenvironment. Analyzing the dining room subenvironment, several activities that could occur in the dining room on a periodic basis are: (a) eating meals, (b) studying/homework, and (c) cleaning. Skills required for eating in the dining room are determined by an analysis of behaviors that are functional and age appropriate for a successful dining experience. One can insure the validity of this analysis by observing a similar situation with nonhandicapped same-aged peers.

How Does a Functional Skills Model Contrast with a Developmental Model?

The functional skills model of habilation contrasts with a developmental model in the following five areas:

Chronological Age

The age of the child or youth is a primary difference between the characteristics and requirements of the two models. A top-down analysis selects behaviors to teach which will be reinforced by the consequences found in the natural environment(s) of the child. As mentioned previously, the habilitative personnel would target for development certain skills for a five-year-old that would be considerably different than those targeted for an adolescent. The peer groups that each of these two handicapped individuals might interact with are widely different. As a result, there are differences in the skills and behaviors that are reinforced. In contrast, a developmental approach largely ignores the requirements of the individual's natural peer group environment. This often leads to targeting skills for development that are age inappropriate.

The need to target age-appropriate skills is illustrated in the following hypothetical example. Teaching an unassertive 18-year-old to be socially assertive in certain interpersonal situations at a work site would be an acceptable intervention. However, this intervention may not be acceptable or may have to be modified somewhat, given the same situation with a five-year-old handicapped boy in the classroom. Teaching assertive behavior to younger children may not produce the same effect on their social environment. The situations that would require (reinforce) assertive behavior in younger children would be a more restricted range of conditions than those for the 18-year old. It is difficult for children to be reinforced for being assertive (even if the child is right) in interpersonal situations with older children or adults while at school. At the very least, it would appear a different form or topography of the response would have to be developed in five-year olds.

In another related illustration, teaching six-year-old handicapped children to clap their hands to elementary songs and riddles is appropriate. Teaching the same skill to handicapped adolescents, using the same types of songs, is age inappropriate. Adolescents express their enjoyment or appreciation for music in a different manner than six-year-old children. They also listen to different kinds of music.

Analyzing Skills to Teach

The functional skills model has been termed a top-down analysis (Brown et al., 1979; Snell, 1983). This indicates that target skills are selected as they relate to requirements of the current or future natural environments. This creates an habilitation plan that is more individualized for the specific needs of the individual. This analysis is conducted from the current and future required skills in the individual's relevant environments. Only those skills that are crucial for the learning of the target (required) skill are taught. Training personnel also entertain any environmental adaptations that will allow the handicapped individual to perform the skill to a degree that would result in the same outcome.

In contrast, a developmental model utilizes a "bottom-up" approach by identifying skills appropriate for the individual's mental age or level. Functional skills may only be targeted later as a function of the learner acquiring skills that are indicative of lower levels of intellectual capability. The outcome of a "bottom-up" analysis can be that a handicapped adolescent may spend much time developing skills appropriate for younger children prior to receiving training on skills that are more appropriate for his or her age.

Training

One of the major problems cited about skill development of handicapped individuals is the lack of generalization of acquired skills across relevant settings, situations, and/or environments. A major tenet of a functional skills model is to train the target behaviors or skills in the environments/subenvironments which reinforce its occurrence whenever possible. It may not always be feasible to train in the target setting. In this case, some of the repertoire can be shaped with a simulation environment in the class or therapy room. This allows the trainer to provide intensive instruction during the development of skills. However, the trainer does not terminate the training until the individual has performed the entire chain of skills in the natural setting(s) correctly. Obviously, this insures the transfer and reinforcement of these skills in the natural context.

In contrast, a developmental model fails to take into account the acquisition and maintenance of targeted skills in relevant settings. Rather, generalization is usually assumed. This assumption is evidenced in the delivery of a variety of therapies of services which are conducted in one to one sessions in an office. Responses are trained to occur in the therapy room to the particular therapist. Often, follow-up in the natural environment is not conducted subsequent to training. This failure to insure that the trained response is being exhibited under natural conditions and situations is a major reason for the lack of durability and generalizability of these trained behaviors.

Assessment

A fourth major difference between the two approaches is in the area of assessment. There is a heavy reliance on criterion-referenced measurement of skills with the functional skills approach, versus norm-referenced measures of behavior. The assessment of behavior should be concerned with the identification of skill(s) that are present and skills which are deficient, to some degree. This method of assessment allows one to directly translate obtained assessment data to targeted objectives. Data are collected only on the skill or skills in question. On the other hand, the utilization of test data from norm-referenced assessment does not lead easily to an analysis of deficient skill(s). The purpose of going from assessment data to training objectives becomes less clear and more difficult. Norm-referenced assessment determines the child's developmental level. Given the mental age, the child is programmed, i.e., all skills relevant for someone of that mental age are targeted. It is assumed that all skills at that level are equally deficient. This can often be an incorrect assumption about handicapped children in that they can have "splinter" skills and abilities.

Teaching Responsibility

In a functional skills model, training should occur to natural situations and stimuli. Therefore, habilitation becomes the responsibility of all people involved with the handicapped child. While the school personnel can assist in identifying relevant objectives for the handicapped child for nonschool personnel, learning is an event that needs to occur in the everyday activities of the child, and directed by people who come in contact with the child in those situations. In contrast, a developmental model primarily focuses on the delivery of instruction from teachers in school classrooms.

How to Conduct a Functional Skills Analysis

The contrast between a functional skills analysis and a developmental model is presented above. The utilization of a functional skills model is particularly important when training personnel consider the needs of older handicapped children, adolescents and youth. The following sequence of activities delineates procedures within a functional skills analysis.

Survey Environment

The first requirement in conducting a functional skills analysis is to identify and survey the target child's or youth's environments and/or subenvironments. The utilization of the four domains specified by Snell (1983) provides a format that insures all relevant areas are identified. Each domain should be analyzed into the different environments, subenvironments, and activities (within each subenvironment). These preliminary activities lead to the identification of skills that are required in the individual's natural environments.

Identify Skills

In identifying skills required for each activity several factors need to be considered. The targeted skills(s) should lead to a level of competence within the target environment/subenvironment. In attempting to identify such skills, a technique termed *social comparison* can be used (Kazdin & Matson, 1981). The trainer identifies skills exhibited by same-aged peers who frequently interact successfully in the environment/subenvironments of concern. These skills, with any needed adaptations, become the target skills. Utilizing the example in a previous section, the dining room subenvironment identified the behavior of eating meals as one activity relevant to that environment. What skills should be trained? The trainer identifies target skills by observing other nonhandicapped individuals interact successfully in a similar dining room situation. Nutter and Reid (1978) utilized social comparison methodology in teaching severely handicapped women to wear appropriate color-coordinated clothing. In identifying what skills should be taught, the authors observed over 600 women in nearby public places. These observations helped them identify what color-coordination patterns (in wearing apparel) would be an acceptable standard.

In addition to identifying target skills, other factors regarding the targeted skills need to be assessed a priori. The timing of a behavior (conditions under which it will occur) as well as the duration of its occurrence can be important factors to consider. Some skills are reinforced if they occur under specific conditions, whereas their occurrence is not reinforced under other conditions. For example, a possible target skill during eating is to wipe the mouth periodically with a napkin. With some foods, the rate of this behavior should be more frequent due to increased spillage. It is important for the individual to discriminate the times (conditions) under which this behavior should occur. Another example of the importance of timing of behavior can be offered. It may be acceptable during mealtimes with relatives to reach for the salt shaker (across table). However, when guests are seated at the table, one usually asks someone to pass the salt to him or her. Conversation at the dinner table can be used to illustrate that duration of occurrence may be just as important as when the behavior occurs in terms of social reinforcement. Appropriate dinner time conversation would be brief, allowing others to speak and thus not dominating the conversation. Training personnel should teach the individual not only the behavior of conversing, but also how to converse for short periods at certain times during the mealtime (e.g., not talking while others are talking).

Snell (1983) identifies a number of these types of training issues in the fluency stage of training. Oftentimes, reinforcement for the occurrence of the behavior in the natural environment depends on training it to a level of fluency that will access such reinforcement.

Another consideration in this phase is the schedule of reinforcement. The behavior needs to be trained to a level of occurrence that "blend-in" with the reinforcement delivery schedule in the post-training environment. Two related factors are the type of consequent events used, and the occurrence (or lack) of any additional prompts in the post-therapy environment. Consideration of reinforcement contingencies operable in the post-training environment is crucial for successful maintenance of new behaviors.

Assess Target Child's Skills

The third activity assesses the target child on these skills identified from the above analysis. The most preferable method of measurement is direct observation. In situations where direct observation may not be feasible, structured role playing may provide data that can approximate direct observation data.

Identify Discrepancies and Select Objectives

The next activity compares the data collected from the previous two activities and identifies the discrepancies between the child's performance and the levels of behaviors or skills needed in a given environment. From this list of discrepancies, training objectives are prioritized and those that require more immediate attention are selected. It is suggested to initially target those skills that allow the individual to function as independently as possible in the shortest period of time (Snell, 1983). If certain prerequisite skills are lacking, then these are identified and selected as training objectives. Criterion levels and other conditions identifying fluency, generality and maintenance are specified in each training objective.

Identify Training Conditions

In this phase, the designer identifies how the training will proceed. Will training be conducted in the natural environment immediately? This is most preferable, if possible. However, in teaching a complex chain of behavior, it is often unfeasible to train in the natural environment with one who has few of the needed skills. Prompting, continuous and frequent reinforcement and massed trials may be needed in order for the child or youth to acquire the set of skills. In these cases, the community environment may not facilitate the operation of a training regimen. If such is the case, simulated conditions might be developed to allow the more rigorous training procedures to be effected.

In teaching handicapped individuals to eat at a fast food restaurant, a simulation was developed to allow skill acquisition in a relatively short period of time (VandenPol, Iwata, Ivancic, Page, Neef, & Whitley, 1981). Simulation training involved responding to the presentation of slides representing various aspects of the restaurant experience and/or role playing a particular interaction with a trainer serving as cashier. Of course, generalization probes were conducted to insure that performance would eventually occur under the natural, targeted conditions.

An additional requirement is to schedule training a priori. Who will train, when will they train, and for how long will they train?

These issues when set a priori insure that the training will be delivered across a period of time.

Identify Possible Adaptations

Finally, any adaptations to the task that can be made which allow a handicapped child to perform a skill more readily needs to be examined. For example, alternate communication systems (communication boards, manual signing, electrical devices) allow handicapped individuals the capability to acquire complex verbal and community skills that might be otherwise unavailable to someone who is nonvocal. Adjusting a functional task to enable performance has been termed the *principal of partial participates* (Snell, 1983).

Once these activities are conducted and a functional analysis of relevant skills is completed, training can be initiated. It is now important to utilize a behavioral technology for training identified relevant skills with handicapped people, as the next section indicates.

TRAINING THROUGH BEHAVIORAL TECHNOLOGY: HOW TO TEACH

The previous section presented a curriculum approach which identifies and trains functional skills for the relevant environment(s). When these are trained to a criterion level, the handicapped individual experiences greater independence in his or her environment. Therefore, the target of training programs should be the development of relevant behaviors that maximize the individual's independence in the least restrictive environment.

A second crucial aspect in the treatment of handicapped children is how training is delivered. This is just as important in maximizing an individual's independence as the targeting of functional skills. The following section presents basic information on general behavioral training/teaching procedures including shaping, prompting and chaining. Contingencies are equally important, if not more so, in developing new behaviors. However, it is assumed that the reader has working knowledge of the utilization of contingencies, and as such, this is not fully discussed.

Elements of the Learning Cycle

How does a child learn to respond? A behavioral view examines the observable elements of the process. Behavior occurs in the presence of stimuli. The behavior is then followed by an environmental event, termed the consequence. A stimulus is an observable event or object that precedes the behavior or response. Behavior (or response) as defined in this context, has to be observable and measurable. Consequences are events that follow behavior, which influence the future probability of the behavior they follow. If, as a result of a consistent consequence, the child's behavior maintains or increases above the previous level, we term this relationship reinforcement. If the child's rate of behavior decreases, as a function of the consequence, then we term this relationship punishment.

When the child's behavior can be reliably predicted given the presence of certain stimuli, the behavior is said to be under stimulus control. Stimulus control is defined as, the highly probable occurrence of a behavior or sets of behaviors in the presence of certain stimuli. A child who will reliably say "shoe" when he has his socks on (and can't find his shoe) demonstrates stimulus control. This set of stimuli reliably evokes the spoken word "shoe." When incorrect responses occur, training procedures are developed to obtain the correct response from the child consistently, given the presence of specific stimuli. Reinforcement for the correct response is provided, while the delivery of reinforcement is withheld for an incorrect response. If this strategy is successful, the child will consistently respond correctly to the stimulus conditions.

The development of many skills is usually more complex than the acquisition of one isolate behavior or response to a stimulus. Rather, most skills are chains or steps of behaviors. A behavioral chain is a sequence of stimuli and responses which leads to the delivery of reinforcement at the completion of the chain (Popovich, 1981). Each step in the chain serves as the discriminative stimulus for the next step or behavior.

The remainder of this chapter will deal with methods to develop new behaviors: shaping, prompting, and chaining techniques. Again, this is not to derogate the role of contingencies in maintaining behavior to a lesser import. As mentioned previously, a working knowledge of reinforcement principles is assumed.

Shaping

With complex community behaviors, a chain of responses will have to be developed gradually. Shaping is the process of reinforcing behavioral approximations to a desired goal. Shaping allows the trainer to build a new behavior or a chain of behaviors by reinforcing gradual approximations to that behavior or chain. In shaping, the trainer progressively alters the behavioral requirements for reinforcement at various phases of the training. This can produce the gradual acquisition of the behavior or chain of behaviors.

The first step in developing a plan to shape behavior is to specify a clear criterion level for reinforcement at each phase of the program. The initial form of the behavior to be reinforced should be specified a priori. This allows anyone conducting the training to deliver reinforcement in a consistent manner. The personnel implementing the training program should not reinforce responses that do not meet the criteria for reinforcement. Then, specification of the gradual successive approximations to be reinforced is needed for programmatic success.

A programmed strategy to increase voice volume in young developmentally delayed children illustrates shaping techniques (Fleece, Gross, O'Brien, Kistner, Rothblum, & Drabman, 1981). This program utilized a sound sensitive apparatus to measure voice volume during a classroom recitation of rhymes exercise. The shaping program consisted of progressive alterations of the sound sensitivity of the apparatus. The illumination of a colorful display through the voice-activated relay was utilized as a reinforcer when the voice volume was of sufficient strengths. This procedure was successful in obtaining successive increments of voice volume during the treatment.

Prompting and Fading Techniques

The use of three different types of prompts makes it much easier to develop complex chains of behaviors. Prompts provide additional cues at points in the behavioral chain where the student's behavior is lacking. Several types and levels of prompts utilized for this purpose are verbal and/or gestural, modeled, and physical prompts. Combined with a time delay fading technique, this training strategy allows the child to eventually perform the step(s) in the chain independently.

Verbal prompts are additional cues (or stimuli) in the form of verbal instructions that indicate to the child the response desired. Verbal prompts can be used with gestural prompts. Gestural prompts can be hand or arm movements, head nods or pointing to an area, which would indicate the desired behavior. Often, these prompts can be presented simultaneously. For example, a teacher could give a verbal prompt such as, "Rinse your hands" while motioning to the child's hand and the water.

Verbal and gestural prompts are the least intrusive types of prompts to use in comparison to the other two types of prompts. Therefore, one wants to provide these to get the desired response prior to using the other two prompts. How to fade verbal and/or gestural prompts as well as other prompts will be discussed in a later section.

Modeled prompts show the child the specific form of the response. An example of a modeled prompt would be the trainer demonstrating how to turn on the water and then providing the child the opportunity to perform this behavior. Modeled prompts are more intrusive than verbal prompts in that they show the child how to behave.

Physical prompts are more commonly used with children and youth having severe handicaps. With physical prompting, the teacher insures that the child will perform the correct response (and thus receive reinforcement). Using the previous illustration of teaching a child to turn on the water, after verbal and modeled prompts failed to obtain this behavior, physical prompting would be used. The trainer would place his or her hand on or over the child's hand and physically guide it to the faucet, guide the child to turn the faucet on, and then provide reinforcement for completing the desired behavior. Physical prompting is the most intrusive type of prompting and therefore should be used only after the previous two types of prompts have failed.

To summarize, prompts allow the trainers to teach complex

chains of behaviors by providing additional stimuli (cues) where needed. Prompts are provided in a manner that allows for the least amount of help (prompt) to be given first. Therefore, the sequence of presentation of prompts is verbal and/or gestural, modeled, and then physical.

The sequence in which these prompts should be faded is the opposite sequence in which they were delivered. The more "intrusive" prompts are faded before other prompts, thereby reducing the number of cues to the student and facilitating independent performance.

There are two methods that can be used to fade prompts. In many instances, both can be used concurrently. The two methods are: (a) providing less of the prompt (until it is completely eliminated) and (b) time delay fading techniques.

In fading physical prompts by reducing the amount of the prompt given, less and less guidance is provided, which allows the child the opportunity to gradually perform more of the motor requirements of the skill. Shadowing is a procedure whereby all physical guidance is gradually removed (Popovich, 1981). At that point the trainer shadows the hand or arm movement of the child, but does not physically touch the child unless needed. When this is effective the trainer then begins to fade the shadowed prompt.

Modeled, verbal, and gestural prompts can also be partially withdrawn. The child will then begin to acquire the skill independently without the use of any prompts which, of course, is the desired condition. For example, the trainer fades a modeled prompt by demonstrating two-thirds of the chain, with the child performing the last third of the chain under less intrusive prompts.

The second fading method, time delay fading, involves gradually increasing the length of time between the presentation of the original stimulus and the prompt stimulus. Time delay has been used more extensively in language training (Halle, Marshall, & Spradlin, 1979; Smeets & Striefel, 1976; Snell & Gast, 1981; Striefel, Bryan, & Aikins, 1974). In utilizing a time delay fading procedure, the prompt is removed by increasing the time between the presentation of the original stimulus and the prompt. As a result, the percentage of times the prompt is needed decreases across the training program until the learner is responding to the original stimulus.

Researchers at the University of Kansas and Kansas Neurological Institute utilized a time delay procedure to teach six severely retarded children to verbally request their food at breakfast and lunch (Halle, Marshall, & Spradlin, 1979). All children were called by staff to a counter. During baseline, the food was delivered to them upon their arrival at the counter. The training strategy time delayed the presentation of the food for 15-seconds after the children arrived at the counter. Three of the six children learned to make an appropriate request as a result of this procedure. The remaining three were provided an additional prompt in addition to the 15-second delay. If the child did not request the food at the end of the 15-second delay, the staff member modeled the appropriate response, "Tray, please!" If the child modeled that response, the tray was given immediately. If the child did not respond correctly, a modeled prompt by the staff member was given twice more. If a correct response was still not forthcoming the tray was then given. This strategy resulted in two of the three children acquiring the spontaneous requesting response. The sixth child required a more intensive training and fading procedure in order to learn to verbally request his food.

Chaining Methods

The previous section illustrated how shaping and prompts can be used to teach handicapped children and adolescents new skills. There are three chaining methods that can be utilized in building a behavioral chain: (a) backward chaining, (b) forward chaining, and (c) graduated guidance. All three methods utilize prompts and time delay techniques to fade prompts in developing large units of behavior (e.g., taking a bath, doing the laundry, tying shoelaces, etc.). These chaining methods differ along the following dimensions: (a) the point(s) in the chain when reinforcement for correct responding is provided, (b) the point(s) where prompts are given and then faded, (c) the selection of the target step(s), and (d) the presentation of part of the task versus the entire task.

In backward chaining, the last step(s) of the sequence are taught first. Prompts are provided on these steps, if needed and subsequently faded. Reinforcement is always delivered after successful completion of the last step of the sequence. As the child demonstrates independent behavior in these latter steps, the steps that occur earlier in the sequence are targeted until the child is performing the entire sequence independently. In backward chaining, the first steps taught are those in the "back of the chain." As the child acquires the end part of the chain, the target steps selected become those in the front of the chain. Backward chaining has been used for a variety of skills and several manuals describing their application to such skills have been developed (Baker, Brightman, Heifetz, & Murphy, 1976; Bensberg, 1965; Watson, 1974a).

Teaching feeding skills to children who do not feed themselves independently is well adapted to backward chaining procedures. Cipani (1981) used a backward chaining method to teach a client to independently self-feed with a spoon. The client was initially physically prompted through all the steps of the behavioral chain, i.e., grasping spoon, bringing spoon to plate, scooping the food, lifting the spoon to mouth, inserting the spoon in mouth, removing the spoon and leaving the food in the mouth (delivery of reinforcement). The physical prompts were then removed from the back of the chain. The trainer was able to develop independent behavior after the client was physically prompted to scoop the food on the spoon. A diet change resulted in complete independence for the entire chain.

In forward chaining, the target step is in the initial part of the chain depending on what steps are already in the child's repertoire. Reinforcement is provided upon the correct response occurring on the target step and often at the end of the sequence.

Forward chaining has been used in training handicapped people to independently perform many skills (Lewis, Fernetti, & Keilitz, 1975; Bender & Valletutti, 1976). A forward chaining procedure would teach the child to independently perform the steps, starting with deficient step(s) in the front part of the sequence. In teaching skills in a forward chaining fashion, verbal and/or modeled prompts are provided prior to providing a physical prompt. Reinforcement would occur upon completion of the targeted step. Prompts are then faded on the training step. Training is conducted until the child is performing this step independently. This process is then implemented for the new target step. This process is continued until the child performs the entire chain (without prompts). Prompts are removed via one or both of the two fading methods, time delay, or prompt reduction.

Graduated guidance is a method that provides guidance wherever needed throughout the entire chain (Azrin & Armstrong, 1973; Azrin, Schaeffer, & Wesolowski, 1976). The child is always reinforced at the completion of the chain. During each training opportunity, fading of previously provided prompts are attempted using time delay techniques. By delaying the prompt at various parts of the chain, the child is gradually taught to independently perform the entire chain. Each step becomes a target step. Graduated guidance is slightly different than the two previous chaining methods in that prompts are delivered and faded as needed (trainer discretion) on all the steps of the chain. The emphasis is on giving a minimal amount of guidance while allowing the child to complete the chain.

The graduated guidance chaining method can be highly effective in teaching handicapped children complex skills. However, it does require more skill and judgement from the trainer than forward or backward chaining. The trainer makes judgements as to when prompts are necessary, during each training opportunity. Trainers who work with this procedure over time develop refined skills in judgement as to when to prompt and when to delay a prompt.

There are a number of varieties of these three basic methods. Most applications of chaining methods involve a graduated series of prompts. In teaching two male adolescents and one male adult seven components of laundry skills, a three-prompt procedure consisting of verbal instruction, modeling, and graduated guidance was used (Thompson, Braam, & Fugua, 1982). Laundry skills were analyzed into sorting, loading washer, setting washer, emptying washer, cleaning lint screen, setting dryer, and starting dryer. There were 74 discrete responses across all seven components. In that respective order, an incorrect or no response resulted in the trainer delivering the next level prompt until the correct response occurred. Each component was trained to 100% accuracy for two consecutive trials and then chained onto the previous learned components for two consecutive correct trials. With this method, the range of sessions needed to reach criterion on all components was 75-92. The follow-up data, 10 months after training, indicated that for two of the subjects, skills were maintained. Additionally, these skills generalized as doing laundry at a public laundromat. The other subject averaged 51% accuracy at follow-up. However, this subject was the only one who had failed to receive the opportunity to practice the skill during the follow-up period.

Another of the chaining strategies has utilized a graduated series of prompts, but also paired verbal instruction with the delivery of more interview prompts. In a study teaching three mending skills (buttons, hems, and seams) to four adolescent males and one adolescent female, Cronin and Cuvo (1979) used the following sequence of prompts: (a) no help, (b) verbal instruction, (c) verbal instruction plus modeling, (d) verbal instruction plus physical guidance, and (e) verbal instruction plus visual cue (this type of prompting available only for stitch length and correcting button position). More structured prompts were provided only after failure to respond correctly to less intrusive prompts within five seconds. All skills were rapidly acquired and maintained at one and two week follow-ups. These skills also generalized to untrained tasks.

A slight adaptation to forward chaining methods is to initially train a part of the total task to criterion and then chain on additional steps. With a partial task method, the trainers would only present the stimuli for the initial (forward chaining) or latter (backward chaining) steps and then just train those parts of the chain. Steps are then added until the entire chain is taught. However, only those steps that are being trained or have been trained are completed during training. An example of a partial task approach with a nine-step handwashing program of a total task forward chaining procedure would be to train the child on the initial target steps (e.g., turning on water, putting hands in) by presenting the initial stimulus ("wash your hands") and delivering the reinforcement after the child puts his hands in. The task is then presented again in the same manner repeatedly.

Partial task approaches are adaptable to teach complex chains of behaviors required for community skills. In summary, a variety of community skills have been trained using shaping and chaining methods, such as self-medication (Brickey, 1978); independent toothbrushing (Horner & Keilitz, 1975); pedestrian skills (Matson, 1980; Page, Iwata, & Neef, 1976); public transportation (Neef, Iwata, & Page, 1978); skills in using a pocket calculator (Smeets,

1978); and ordering a meal at a restaurant (Marholin, O'Toole, Touchette, Berger, & Doyle, 1979).

SUMMARY

The previous article identified a special technology for exceptional children and adolescents. It has implications for what is taught as well as how it is taught. Particularly with older children and adolescents, skills that are functional in the natural environments should be selected and targeted for intervention. These skills, once developed, will allow the individual to integrate to his or her fullest extent possible in the mainstream of society.

The use of behavioral training techniques by training personnel allows the handicapped individual to acquire skills which he or she may have failed to learn through observation alone. The use of contingencies is inherent in any sound behavioral training paradigm. However, to develop new skills, shaping and chaining techniques will be needed as well to train successfully such skills to criterion. There are a variety of techniques to develop complex chains of behavior required in community settings. Prompts, and fading of those prompts, will be used to get the correct form of the behavior occurring so it can be reinforced.

As handicapped children and adolescents more frequently transition to least restrictive community sites, both sets of instructional technology will be essential to achieve successful transition. Teaching functional skills, through behavioral technology, will allow more people to live a useful, productive life.

REFERENCES

Azrin, H. H., & Armstrong, P. M. (1973). "The Mini-meal": A method for teaching eating skills to the profoundly retarded. *Mental Retardation, 11*, 9-11.

Azrin, H. H., Schaeffer, R. M., & Wesolowski, M. D. (1976). A rapid method of teaching profoundly and retarded persons to dress. *Mental Retardation, 14*, 29-33.

Baker, B. L., Brightman, A. J., Heifetz, L. J., & Murphy, D. M. (1976). *Steps to independence: A skills training series for children with special needs.* Champaign, IL: Research Press.

Bender, M., & Valletutti, P. J. (1976). *Teaching the moderately and severely handicapped: Curriculum objectives, strategies and activities*. Baltimore: University Park Press.

Bensberg, G. J. (1965). *Teaching the mentally retarded: Handbook for ward personnel*. Atlanta: Southern Regional Educational Board.

Brickey, M. A. (1978). A behavioral procedure for teaching self-medication. *Mental Retardation, 16*, 29-32.

Brown, L., Branston, M. B., Baumgart, D., Vincent, L., Falvey, M., & Schroeder, J. (1979). Using the characteristics of current and subsequent least restrictive environment as factors in the development of curricular content for severely handicapped students. *AAESPH Review, 4*, 407-424.

Cipani, E. (1981). Contingency and ecological components in training a profoundly retarded adult to self-feed. *Behavioral Engineering, 7*, 23-26.

Cronin, K. A., & Cuvo, A. J. (1979). Teaching mending skills to mentally retarded adolescents. *Journal of Applied Behavior Analysis, 12*, 401-406.

Fleece, L., Gross, A., O'Brien, T., Kistner, J., Rothblum, E., & Drabman, R. (1981). Elevation of voice volume in young developmentally delayed children via an operant shaping procedure. *Journal of Applied Behavior Analysis, 14*, 351-355.

Halle, J. W., Marshall, A. M., & Spradlin, J. E. (1979). Time delay: A technique to increase language use and facilitate generalization in retarded children. *Journal of Applied Behavior Analysis, 12*, 431-439.

Horner, D. R., & Keilitz, I. (1975). Training mentally retarded adolescents to brush their teeth. *Journal of Applied Behavior Analysis, 8*, 301-309.

Kazdin, A. E., & Matson, J. L. (1981). Social validation in mental retardation. *Applied Research in Mental Retardation, 2*, 39-53.

Lewis, P. J., Fernetti, C. L., & Keilitz, I. (1975). *Use of deodorant*. Parsons, KS: Project MORE.

Marholin, II, D., O'Toole, K. M., Touchette, P. E., Berger, P. L., & Doyle, D. A. (1979). "I'll have a Big Mac, large fries, large Coke, and apple pie" or teaching adaptive community skills. *Behavior Therapy, 10*, 236-248.

Matson, J. L. (1980). A controlled group study of pedestrian skill training for the mentally retarded. *Behavior Research and Therapy, 18*, 99-106.

Neef, N. A., Iwata, B., & Page, T. (1978). Public transportation training: In vivo versus classroom instruction. *Journal of Applied Behavior Analysis, 11*, 331-344.

Nutter, D., & Reid, D. H. (1978). Teaching retarded women a clothing selection skill using community norms. *Journal of Applied Behavior Analysis, 11*, 475-487.

Page, T. J., Iwata, B. A., & Neef, N. A. (1976). Teaching pedestrian skills to retarded persons. Generalization from the classroom to the natural environment. *Journal of Applied Behavior Analysis, 9*, 433-444.

Popovich, D. (1981). *Effective educational and behavioral programming for severely and profoundly handicapped students: A manual for teachers and aides*. Baltimore: Paul H. Brookes.

Smeets, P. M. (1978). Teaching retarded adults monetary skills using an experimental calculator. *Behavioral Engineering, 5*, 51-59.

Smeets, P. H., & Striefel, S. (1976). Acquisition of sign reading by transfer of stimulus control in a deaf retarded girl. *Journal of Mental Deficiency Research, 20*, 197-205.

Snell, M. E. (1983). *Systematic instruction of the moderately and severely handicapped*. (2nd Edition) Columbus, OH: Charles E. Merrill Publishing Co.

Snell, M. E., & Gast, D. L. (1981). Applying time delay procedure to the instruction of the severely handicapped. *The Journal of the Association for the Severely Handicapped, 6*, 3-14.

Striefel, S., Bryan, K. S., & Aikins, D. A. (1974). Transfer of stimulus control from motor to verbal stimuli. *Journal of Applied Behavior Analysis, 7*, 123-135.

Thompson, T. J., Braam, S. J., & Fugua, R. W. (1982). Training and generalization of laundry skills: A multiple probe evaluation with handicapped persons. *Journal of Applied Behavior Analysis, 15*, 177-182.

VandenPol, R. A., Iwata, B. A., Ivancic, M. T., Page, T. J., Neef, N. A., & Whitley, F. P. (1981). Teaching the handicapped to eat in public places: Acquisition, generalization and maintenance of restaurant skills. *Journal of Applied Behavior Analysis, 14*, 61-69.

Watson, L. S. (1974a). *A manual for teaching behavior modification skills to staff: An inservice training program for parents, teachers, nurses and relevant direct care staff*. Libertyville, IL: Behavior Modification Technology.

Watson, L. S. (1974b). *Training proficiency scale: An assessment instrument for evaluating behavior modification training proficiency of staff*. Libertyville, IL: Behavior Modification Technology.

SECTION III:
THEORY, RESEARCH, AND PRACTICE

Teaching and Training Relevant Community Skills to Mentally Retarded Persons

Johnny L. Matson

ABSTRACT. The development of methods to enhance the quality of life for the handicapped has progressed rapidly in recent years. The current paper provides a review of some of the major teaching and training developments that have occurred in this connection. The range of topics addressed reflects present developments in teaching community skills to persons with mental retardation as well as changes that are likely to occur in the next few years.

One of the major changes in the habilitation of the handicapped in recent years has been the move away from large, congregate institutions to smaller, community-based residential facilities (Matson & Mulick, 1983). This trend has had many ramifications, not only for handicapped persons themselves, but also for the professionals who are responsible for their care and personal growth.

In particular, the decision to integrate handicapped individuals into the community has been a challenge for educators and psychologists, for several reasons. First, there was until very recently, no well defined technology to teach the skills that handicapped persons would need to be able to cope in community-based living arrangements. This was particularly problematic in the case of older persons, many of whom had spent the majority of their lives in

Johnny L. Matson is affiliated with the Department of Psychology, Louisiana State University, Baton Rouge, LA 70803-5501.

institutions where such pedestrian skills as cooking, balancing a checkbook, and so on were not necessary. Second, many handicapped persons had been placed in institutions for very aberrant behavior: extreme aggression, schizophrenia, manic depressive psychosis, and other serious interpersonal problems. With the recent emphasis on community placement, a much stronger and more sophisticated approach to enhancing adaptive behavior was needed. Third, community placement requires much higher levels of competence in social/interpersonal behavior, given the importance of these responses to facilitate acceptance in the community. All these factors necessitated much stronger and more sophisticated methods of assessment and treatment. While the current state of affairs is far from optimal, major advances have been made. These technological innovations are the focus of this paper.

The procedures to be described are applicable for young and old in school settings and community residences such as group homes, including a wide range of intellectual levels that are represented among persons with mental retardation. It should be pointed out that the orientation of the paper is based on learning principles associated with behavior modification, because behavioral applications are the only methods and treatments that currently have empirical support.

The subject matter of the field has been defined by the research efforts of professionals in education and psychology. For this review, the research has been divided into four broad areas: independence in the home setting; transportation and leisure; interpersonal skills; and a description of overall impressions and potential areas for further advances. The topic of independence in the home concentrates on dressing, maintaining a living environment, preparing meals and other elements that enhance individuals' abilities to care for themselves. The transportation and leisure section provides a discussion of research on such abilities as pedestrian and shopping skills, as well as a review of studies that have been conducted to enhance handicapped persons' abilities to spend free time in constructive and useful ways. A discussion of the training of interpersonal skills in mentally retarded individuals, which has received a great deal of attention in recent years, follows.

ADAPTIVE SKILLS

There are a wide variety of behaviors which are of importance in enhancing independent living. A developmental, evolutionary approach will be followed here, beginning with the most rudimentary problems and moving from there to the discussion of more complex skills. Less complex skills (e.g., toileting, eating, dressing) have most typically been treated with operant conditioning, whereas more complex behaviors have been treated with a wider variety of techniques, including self-control procedures, modeling, and other social learning methods. The skills to be covered include toileting; eating, dressing and personal hygiene; community survival; and vocational and social skills.

Toileting

The problem of continence is a frequent and difficult one among persons with handicaps, particularly individuals with mental retardation. Historically, failure to acquire diurnal continence, in particular, was sufficient to preclude the development of other, more advanced skills. Until recently, the resolution of this problem was considered impossible. Thus, these persons were doomed to a life of constant hospitalization, receiving minimal amounts of food and shelter and no training. The advent of effective toilet training methods had the impact of freeing these persons for less restricted, more habilitative lives. In addition, early studies in this field clearly demonstrated that even very recalcitrant, problematic individuals could be effectively trained. The momentum created by toilet training research led to an optimistic climate and extensive work that created a virtual explosion of new knowledge on training adaptive community skills.

The earliest studies on toilet training were conducted by Ellis (1963). One study used a very simple program of reinforcing appropriate episodes of toileting. It proved to be very effective, as was demonstrated by Dyan (1964) at the same facility for the mentally retarded in Louisiana.

The training model of providing "setting events" followed by reinforcement of appropriate responses and punishment of inappropriate responses has become a common and effective method. Setting events involve the following components: prompting the handicapped person to go to the toilet, placing the person on a commode at regular intervals, having staff available to assist with toileting when self-initiations occur, training verbal skills (so the person can more readily report the need to void), and training disrobing skills needed for independent toileting.

Among studies that followed was one reported by Giles and Wolf (1966) that exemplifies the research of that period. They treated five severely retarded children throughout their waking hours over a 60 day period. Various reinforcers were used when appropriate toileting behavior occurred, together with aversive stimuli in the form of temporarily withheld meals. The results indicated that three children were independently initiating appropriate toileting behavior at close to 100% levels (without soiling episodes), while the other two showed major improvement. Studies such as this one and the report of Dyan (1964) demonstrated that these skills could be trained.

This research solved the basic question of identifying an effective method(s) to train toileting skills. More recently, as with most self-help research, studies have evolved to a more complex level. Issues of generalization, maintenance of treatment gains, and rapidity of treatment effects are examples of variables currently receiving increased research attention.

To assist in identifying diurnal episodes of socially undesirable voiding, technology has been brought to bear, such as the pants alarm apparatus developed by Azrin, Bugle, and O'Brien (1971). This equipment is similar to a device described by Van Wagenen and Murdock (1966). The device, which is sensitive to moisture, buzzes when the wearer urinates or defecates in his or her clothes. A second, similar device sounds when persons void in the toilet. While this idea would seem to be an appealing one, it has not caught on and has rarely been reported in research since its initial invention. Similarly, having visited many programs for the handicapped around the country, this author is not aware of widespread clinical use of these devices. It is likely that persons being monitored with the apparatus pull it off or otherwise incapacitate it by plan or just through moving around. Thus, it may not be as practical as was once thought.

The amount of research done on diurnal toileting has slowed greatly. Azrin and colleagues at Anna State Hospital in Illinois did most of the empirically sound research in this area. When they finished their efforts in this field, other researchers did not continue to develop such methods. While more work in this area is needed, further research developments may be limited as a result of the practical utility of existing, tested methods combined with the difficulty of conducting this type of research.

Nocturnal enuresis

The other type of research in this area has applied to nocturnal enuresis. More has been done on this topic, perhaps due to the fact that it is a much more common problem than diurnal enuresis and encopresis. The first major breakthrough in this area was made by Mowrer and Mowrer (1938). This method, still widely used, involves a urine detection device that, when triggered, results in a loud buzz that wakes the child. The idea is to teach the child to respond more quickly to bladder signals to void. This learning-based paradigm has been successfully documented in a number of experimental studies. The research on this approach, while dormant for some time, has been quite plentiful and supportive in recent years. A review of 12 studies since 1965 (Doleys, 1977) indicates that, on the average, bedwetting is initially arrested in about 75% of children treated with an average duration of treatment ranging from 5 to 12 weeks.

Another popular method is called dry-bed training (Azrin, Sneed, & Foxx, 1974). This approach uses the Mowrer and Mowrer bell and pad but adds an intensive, all-night program. The enuretic child is given training in rapid awakening and practice in withholding urine. It requires the child to help clean up accidents, using an overcorrection procedure. Typical of research with this latter method is the work of Bollard, Nettlebeck and Roxbee (1982), who reported a two-year follow-up of 35 children treated with the Mowrer pad or dry-bed training methods. After subjects exhibited 14 consecutive dry nights, the follow-up data over a two-year period indicated only a 41% relapse for each group.

While both of these methods proved to be effective, it is argued that the Mowrer and Mowrer procedure may be the more practical of the two; the dry-bed method requires an inordinately longer time during sleeping hours to implement, at least for the first few days of the program. Given the more feasible implementation program required by Mowrer and Mowrer, its utilization in the intended fashion seems more likely. Furthermore, empirical data exist to support the contention that parents are more favorably disposed toward using the bell and pad which does not require them to remain awake for the majority of the night (Fincham & Spettell, 1984).

More research, particularly with mentally retarded and sensorily handicapped persons, is greatly needed, since the available research has largely been with children who do not have these additional problems. The success of training with mentally retarded adults is particularly questionable, because adults are likely to have been engaging in the inappropriate behavior for a far longer period of time, making effective treatment even more unlikely.

Eating, Dressing, and Personal Hygiene

Assuming that some progress can be made on toileting problems, another area that needs attention is making oneself as physically presentable as possible. Considerable research in social psychology has been done to confirm that appearance is very important in how others are likely to perceive the individual. To insure the greatest likelihood of acceptance in the community, attention to this issue is most certainly required. This topic has been a popular one and has resulted in numerous curricula and research (Reid, 1983). In fact, this is certainly one of the best documented of the skill areas to date.

Teaching independent eating skills has been well-documented in research. Much of the research has involved the reinforcement of very rudimentary skills such as getting food successfully into the mouth. Typical of these efforts is the mini-meal program (O'Brien, Bugle, & Azrin, 1972). With this approach, the eating sequence is broken into small steps. The trainer physically guides the students through the stages of self-feeding, using the least amount of physical guidance necessary to insure proper performance of the skill.

More advanced eating skills are, of course, needed for maximum community integration. There have been several studies performed to address this issue. One effort of this type is described by Matson, Ollendick, and Adkins (1980). This procedure was deemed to be favorable, since no aversive components existed in the program. Training included a three-month program across five levels of performance based on skill level. The broad areas for training included teaching independent eating as well as teaching such collateral socially acceptable behaviors as orderliness, utensil usage, neatness, and table manners. Targeting eating as well as social skills involved in the mealtime setting had the potential of making the 80 mentally retarded adults studied more ready candidates for community placement.

The positive training program, which was referred to as *independence training*, was useful and effective in teaching this wide range of skills. Among the techniques used were modeling, social reinforcement, role playing, and feedback by self and peers. Another study of this type was reported by Marholin, O'Toole, Touchette, Berger, and Doyle (1979). They taught successful skills in ordering and eating in a local McDonald's. Along the same lines, Matson (1979) has described a program to teach mildly and moderately mentally retarded adults to prepare meals independently.

The data suggest that, at least with mild and moderately mentally retarded persons, a wide variety of socially appropriate eating skills can be taught. The more recent studies have emphasized family style dining or dining out where socially appropriate eating is as important as the act of getting the food from the plate to the mouth. Even more recent research with profoundly mentally retarded persons has stressed desirable community skills: using a napkin, helping to clear the table (Wilson, Reid, Phillips, & Burgio, 1984), and bringing food to the mouth with a minimal amount of food spillage (Cipani, 1981).

Another adaptive skill area receiving attention is dressing. Among the skills that have been trained are putting on and removing socks, shoes, and pants (Minge & Ball, 1967; King & Turner, 1975) and selecting clothing that is color coordinated (Nutter & Reid, 1978). In another important adaptive skill area, self-administration of medication, Brickey (1978) taught 20 handicapped men and women in a sheltered workshop to pick up and take their pills at noon from the secretary in the office of the workshop.

Community Survival

A more extensively studied area has been money management. Several authors have indicated that this skill is a very important one for community integration (e.g., McCarver & Craig, 1974). The majority of the work in money management has been done by Cuvo and associates. They have taught mentally retarded persons to sum coins (Lowe & Cautela, 1976) and to determine coin equivalence (Trace, Cuvo, & Criswell, 1977). More recently, a calculator has been used to teach other summative monetary information (Smeets, 1978).

Another pragmatic skill, somewhat related to making change, is telling time. Smeets, Lancioni and Lieshout (1985) worked with four mentally retarded children ages 7.5 to 12, in the mild to moderately retarded range. While the children were not taught the concept of time, they were able to provide verbal responses to visually trained cues. The development of this skill has many important implications for independent living in our society.

Reaction to fire situations is also of extreme importance for those being prepared for community placement. In recent years, fires have claimed the lives of many handicapped persons. Some of these incidents have received a great deal of national attention, such as a fire in Bradley Beach, New Jersey that killed 23 developmentally disabled persons. The first effort to develop a training program to teach such handicapped people to escape from fires was reported by Matson (1980). Through modeling and active rehearsal, subjects were effectively trained to escape their home in case of fire. Another approach which may have considerable potential has been described by Bertch, Fox, and Kwiecinski (1984). Their procedure includes working with both clients and staff as well as making safety checks of the buildings to insure the most fire resistant habitat. They also suggest areas for further investigation.

A wide number of other skills have also been studied empirically. It is not possible in the present paper to give details on all the topics that have received attention, but some samples will be provided to give the reader a better idea of the state of the art. Mobility skills, for example, have been taught as a method of enhancing independent living. The subject of the study was a profoundly mentally retarded person who was wheelchair-bound but could walk with the support of a table or other physical object. With the training provided, she was able to get out of her wheelchair and stand, without prompting, with the help of support from a table or other stable object.

Another interesting area is the training of telephone answering skills. The first study of this type was reported by Matson (1982). In this study, the proper response to a caller and related social amenities were trained. The interest in this area was further demonstrated by Karen, Astin-Smith, and Creasy (1985), who taught several telephone related skills to the mentally retarded persons including calling someone to the phone, referring the caller to another number in case of a wrong number and taking a message from the caller. For the latter two skills, operant and social learning procedures were effectively combined.

Still another topic is community mobility, such as appropriate use of pedestrian skills (Matson, 1980) and ability to ride a bus effectively (Robinson, Griffith, McComish, & Swasbrook, 1984). In the latter study, the subjects learned to locate the bus stop, to board and ride the bus, and to leave the bus. These are skills that are fairly complex, and the ability to teach them to persons from the normal to profoundly mentally retarded range is impressive.

A final example of the development of training programs for advanced community skills is in the area of menstrual care. Richman, Reiss, Bauman, and Bailey (1984), in their successful, behaviorally-based treatment study of this problem, assert that the inability to handle menstrual care by one's self can require a highly aversive duty of staff and/or family. They suggest that particular to this problem is the accompanying body odor which can result in restrictive placement in the community if not trained to a competent level of care.

Leisure activities, an expression of normal development and integration, have likewise begun to receive some attention. In a recent study targeting leisure activity, 214 adolescents characterized as severely mentally retarded were studied (Jeffree & Chesadine, 1984). Leisure activities were primarily passive and solitary. When other activities, a game in this case, were taught, the frequency of active leisure time and social interactions increased. Similarly, independent play greatly increased for severely handicapped adolescents in one study (Meyer, Evans, Wuerch, & Brennan, 1985). In another study, dancing was taught to four severely and profoundly mentally retarded adults (Lagomarcino, Reid, Ivancic, & Faw, 1984). The skills were taught in separate components, consisting of leg movements, arm movements, and coordinated leg and arm movements. Competence was achieved, although some supervision from staff was needed. The authors argued that these dancing skills would enhance normalized activity in the community. Obviously, these and related self-help problems are critical issues in successful community placement, and their modification and or improvement can be very helpful in insuring proper community integration.

Vocational and Social Skills

Two other areas that have begun to receive considerable attention are vocational and social skills training. The former is of great importance, since work is the major activity outside the home for most adults; normalization would dictate that this area also be given considerable attention with the handicapped. On the other hand, social skills have been linked with a wide variety of issues and problems with the handicapped and nonhandicapped alike. Although these two areas currently receive a great deal of attention, it will be possible to give only a brief overview here. The interested reader is referred to Andrasik and Matson (1985) and Rusch (in press) for extensive reviews of these topics.

The vocational literature has expanded at a very rapid rate in recent years. Until recently, the data that were available dealt almost exclusively with sheltered workshop employment. Some researchers have gone so far as to suggest that more sophisticated vocational training was nonexistent 10 years ago (Irvin, Russell, & Heiry, 1984). Typical of early research in this area is the work of Gold and Barclay (1973), whose study dealt with the teaching of visual discriminations in the assembly of bicycle brakes. Similarly, Jackson (1979) taught adult mentally retarded persons to cut chain links.

The early success of this type of training and the emphasis on normalization has led to goals of economic independence and competitive employment (Whitehead, 1979). Thus, more recent efforts have involved training the handicapped to be bus-persons in a full service community restaurant (Certo, Mezzullo, & Hunter, 1985) and increasing work performance by insuring that handicapped persons engaged in competitive employment attend work on a regular basis (Martin, Rusch, Tines, Brulle, & White, 1985). This trend toward more normalized working conditions is most likely to continue for some time to come, and it is, without a doubt, one of the most positive developments that has occurred in the habilitation of the adult handicapped in recent years.

A final area to be reviewed and one that is receiving a considerable amount of attention in recent years is social skills. Poor social adjustment has been found to occur at disproportionately high rates among juvenile delinquents (Roff, Sells, & Golden, 1972). It also has been found to result in increased mental health problems (Cowen, Pederson, Babigian, Izzo, & Trost, 1973) and is considered a defining characteristic of mental retardation (Grossman, 1977). Matson (1980) has noted that the problems of the hard-core, refractory, chronic, mental health patients and those of the mentally retarded are similar; they are social-interpersonal in nature.

Skills that have typically been trained include conversational skills (Matson, 1979); toy play (Berry & Marshall, 1978); lowered levels of talking loudly and "pestering" staff (Matson & Earnhart, 1981); and appropriateness in content of speech, number of words spoken, eye contact, facial expression, and motor movements (Matson, Kazdin, & Esveldt-Dawson, 1980). A variety of training procedures have been used and found to be effective. Researchers in the field view social skills research as having important ramifications for a variety of community activities, including being effective in school and at work (Rusch, in press). The importance of this area for successful community adjustment probably accounts, in part, for the considerable amount of attention it currently receives and which seems likely to continue in the years to come.

SUMMARY

In this paper, an effort has been made to cover some of the areas in which community adaptation skills have been effectively trained. The number of studies in this area has expanded rapidly of late, and the breadth of topics covered is most impressive. It is quite likely that research of this type will continue to be conducted at an ever increasing rate. These data and the research soon to follow should greatly enhance the quality of life for handicapped people.

REFERENCES

Andrasik, F., & Matson, J. L. (1985). Social skills with the mentally retarded. In M. A. Milan & L. L'Abate (Eds.), *Handbook of social skills training and research*. New York: John Wiley and Sons.

Azrin, N. H., Bugle, C., & O'Brien, F. (1971). Behavioral engineering: Two apparatuses for toilet training retarded children. *Journal of Applied Behavior Analysis, 4*, 249-252.

Azrin, N. H., Sneed, T. J., & Foxx, R. M. (1974). Dry-bed training: Rapid elimination of childhood enuresis. *Behaviour Research and Therapy, 12*, 147-156.

Bertch, G., Fox, C. J., & Kwiecinski, J. (1984). Teaching developmentally disabled persons how to react to fires. *Applied Research in Mental Retardation, 5*, 483-497.

Bollard, J. (1982). A 2-year follow-up of bedwetters treated by dry-bed training and standard conditioning. *Behaviour Research and Therapy, 20*, 571-580.

Bollard, J., Nettlebeck, T., & Roxbee, L. (1982). Dry-bed training for childhood bedwetting: A comparison of group with individually administered parent instructions. *Behaviour Research and Therapy, 20*, 209-218.

Brickey, M. A. (1978). A behavioral procedure for teaching self-medication. *Mental Retardation, 16*, 29-32.

Certo, N., Mezzullo, K., & Hunter, D. (1985). The effect of total task chain training on the acquisition of busperson job skills at a full service community restaurant. *Education and Training of the Mentally Retarded, 20*, 148-156.

Cipani, E. (1981). Modifying food spillage in an institutionalized retarded client. *Journal of Behavior Therapy and Experimental Psychiatry, 12*, 261-265.

Doleys, D. M. (1977). Behavioural treatments for nocturnal enuresis in children: A review of the recent literature. *Psychological Bulletin, 84*, 30-54.

Duker, P. C. (1983). Determinants of diurnal bladder control with institutionalized mentally retarded individuals. *American Journal of Mental Deficiency, 87*, 606-610.

Ellis, N. R. (1963). Toilet training the severely defective patient: An S-R reinforcement analysis. *American Journal of Mental Deficiency, 68*, 98-103.

Fincham, F. D., & Spettell, C. (1984). The acceptability of dry bed training and urine alarm training as treatments of nocturnal enuresis. *Behavior Therapy, 15*, 388-394.

Giles, D. K., & Wolf, M. M. (1966). Toilet training institutionalized, severe retardates: An application of operant behavior modification techniques. *American Journal of Mental Deficiency, 70,* 766-780.

Gold, M., & Barclay, C. R. (1973). The learning of difficult visual discrimination by the moderately and severely retarded. *Mental Retardation, 11,* 9-11.

Irvin, L. K., Gersten, R. M., & Heiry, T. J. (1984). Validating vocational assessment of severely mentally retarded persons: Issues and an application. *American Journal of Mental Deficiency, 88,* 411-417.

Jackson, G. M. (1979). The use of visual orientation feedback to facilitate attention and task performance. *Mental Retardation, 17,* 281-284.

Jeffree, D. M., & Chesadine, S. E. (1984). Programmed leisure intervention and the interaction patterns of severely mentally retarded adolescents: A pilot study. *American Journal of Mental Deficiency, 88,* 619-624.

Karen, R. L., Astin-Smith, S., & Creasy, D. (1985). Teaching telephone-answering skills to mentally retarded adults. *American Journal of Mental Deficiency, 89,* 595-609.

King, L. W., & Turner, R. D. (1975). Teaching a profoundly retarded adult at home by non-professionals. *Journal of Behavior Therapy and Experimental Psychiatry, 6,* 117-121.

Lagomarcino, A., Reid, D. H., Ivancic, M. T., & Faw, G. D. (1984). Leisure-dance instruction for severely and profoundly retarded persons: Teaching an intermediate community-living skill. *Journal of Applied Behavior Analysis, 17,* 71-84.

Lowe, M. L., & Cuvo, A. J. (1976). Teaching coin summation to the mentally retarded. *Journal of Applied Behavior Analysis, 9,* 81-87.

Marholin, D., O'Toole, K. M., Touchette, P. E., Berger, P. L., & Doyle, D. A. (1979). "I'll have a Big Mac, large fries, large coke and apple pie," . . . or teaching adaptive community skills. *Behavior Therapy, 10,* 236-248.

Martin, J. E., Rusch, F. R., Tines, J. J., Brulle, A. R., & White, D. M. (1985). Work attendance in competitive employment: Comparison between employees who are nonhandicapped and those who are mentally retarded. *Mental Retardation, 23,* 142-147.

Matson, J. L. (1980). A control group study of pedestrian skills training for the mentally retarded. *Behaviour Research and Therapy, 18,* 99-106.

Matson, J. L. (1979). A field tested system of training meal preparation skills to the retarded. *British Journal of Mental Subnormality, 25,* 14-18.

Matson, J. L. (1982). Independence training versus modeling procedures for teaching phone conversational skills to the mentally retarded. *Behaviour Research and Therapy, 20,* 505-512.

Matson, J. L. (1980). Preventing home accidents: A training program for the retarded. *Behaviour Modification, 4,* 397-410.

Matson, J. L., & Mulick, J. A. (1983). *Handbook of mental retardation.* New York: Pergamon Press.

Matson, J. L., Ollendick, T. H., & Adkins, J. (1980). A comprehensive dining program for mentally retarded adults. *Behaviour Research and Therapy, 18,* 107-112.

McCarver, R. B., & Craig, E. M. (1974). Placement of the retarded in the community: Prognosis and outcome. In N. R. Ellis (Ed.), *International review of research in mental retardation* (Vol. 7). New York: Academic Press.

Meyer, L. H., Evans, I. M., Wuerch, B. B., & Brennan, J. M. (1985). Monitoring the collateral effects of leisure skill instruction: A case study in multiple-baseline methodology. *Behaviour Research and Therapy, 23,* 127-138.

Minge, M. R., & Ball, T. S. (1967). Teaching of self-help skills to profoundly retarded patients. *American Journal of Mental Deficiency, 71,* 864-868.

Mowrer, O. H., & Mowrer, W. M. (1938). Enuresis — A method for its study and treatment. *American Journal of Orthopsychiatry, 8,* 436-459.

Nutter, D., & Reid, D. H. (1978). Teaching retarded women a clothing selection skill using community norms. *Journal of Applied Behavior Analysis, 11,* 475-487.

O'Brien, F., Bugle, C., & Azrin, N. H. (1972). Training and maintaining a retarded child's proper eating. *Journal of Applied Behavior Analysis, 5,* 67-72.

Reid, D. H. (1983). Trends and issues in behavioral research on training feeding and dressing skills. In J. L. Matson & F. Andrasik (Eds.), *Treatment issues and innovations in mental retardation.* New York: Plenum Press.

Richman, G. S., Reiss, M. L., Bauman, K. E., & Bailey, J. S. (1984). Teaching menstrual care to mentally retarded women: Acquisition, generalization and maintenance. *Journal of Applied Behaviour Analysis, 17,* 441-451.

Robinson, D., Griffith, J., McComish, K., & Swasbrook, K. (1984). Bus training for developmentally disabled adults. *American Journal of Mental Deficiency, 89,* 37-43.

Rusch, F. R. (Ed.) (in press). *Competitive employment service delivery models, Methods and issues.* Baltimore: Paul H. Brooks Publishers.

Smeets, P. M. (1978). Teaching retarded adults monetary skills using an experimental calculator. *Behavioral Engineering, 5,* 51-59.

Smeets, P. M., Lancioni, G. E., & Van Lieshout, R. W. (1985). Teaching mentally retarded children to use an experimental device for telling time and meeting appointments. *Applied Research in Mental Retardation, 6,* 51-70.

Trace, M. W., Cuvo, A. J., & Criswell, J. L. (1977). Teaching coin equivalence to the mentally retarded. *Journal of Applied Behavior Analysis, 10,* 85-92.

Van Wagenen, R. K., & Murdock, E. E. (1966). A transistorized signal-package for toilet training of infants. *Journal of Experimental Child Psychology, 3,* 312-314.

Walker, R. I., & Vogelsberg, R. T. (1985). Increasing independent mobility skills for a woman who was severely handicapped and nonambulatory. *Applied Research in Mental Retardation, 6,* 173-184.

Whitehead, C. (1979). Sheltered workshops in the decade ahead: Work and wages, or welfare. In G. T. Bellamy, G. O'Connor, & O. C. Karen (Eds.),

Vocational rehabilitation of severely handicapped persons. Baltimore: University Park Press.

Wilson, P. G., Reid, D. H., Phillips, J. F., & Burgio, L. D. (1984). Normalization of institutional mealtimes for profoundly retarded persons: Effects and noneffects of teaching family-style dining. *Journal of Applied Behavior Analysis, 17,* 189-201.

Research and Practice in Three Areas of Social Competence: Social Assertion, Interviewing Skills, and Conversational Ability

Ennio Cipani

ABSTRACT. Authors of applied research on social competence have generally concentrated on three areas: social assertion, interviewing skills, and conversational ability. Researchers and practitioners hold some similar and some different perspectives regarding a number of methodological variables within this literature. These studies are reviewed, and conclusions are offered about areas of strengths and future research needs and trends.

Social competence has a direct relationship with successful maintenance in community placements (Charles & McGrath, 1962). The importance of developing a training technology to remediate social skills deficiencies is seen in the side effects produced by the absence of social competence. Children deficient in social skills have a high incidence of peer-rejection (Ballard, Corman, Gottlieb, & Kaufman, 1977; Gottlieb, 1975), delinquency (Roff, Seels, & Golden, 1972), and social failure (Bornstein, Bellack, & Hersen, 1977). It is essential that a series of papers on transitioning handicapped children and youth in the community address the development and training of social competence. Research seems to indicate that these children do not simply "out grow" these deficits in social

Ennio Cipani is affiliated with the Department of Special Education, University of the Pacific, Stockton, CA 95211. The author wishes to thank Dr. Floyd O'Brien and Ms. Linda Adams for their helpful comments on earlier drafts of the manuscript.

training competence (Kagan & Moss, 1962). Therefore, the development of a training technology to treat such deficiencies for children and adolescents transitioning to more mainstream community sites is of high priority.

Social competence is not a unitary set of behaviors. Rather, competence should be defined as a function of the specific interpersonal situation (Combs & Slaby, 1977). It is a social judgement about the general quality of an individual's performance in a given situation (Hops, 1983). This paper takes that view by presenting three specific different areas of social competence: social assertion, interviewing skills, and conversational ability. Each of these areas pinpoints specific interpersonal situations where the presence of certain skills or behavior would lead to a competent successful interaction in the specific situation. There are many more areas involving social skills and competence, but to do justice to the research and training concerns in these areas, the focus is necessarily restricted. Research reviewed focused on the treatment and remediation of skills with handicapped children or youth. When relevant, landmark studies with other clinical populations are discussed. Practical concerns within each area, from the standpoint of application in natural settings are presented.

The research within each interpersonal area is reviewed as to the studies' adherence to a number of methodological variables. The current status and future research needs with regard to the specific variable is presented, where applicable. Finally, practical concerns in developing such a skill with respect to training strategies, assessment, generalization, and validation of treatment effects are presented.

SOCIAL ASSERTION

Subjects and Setting

The majority of subjects used to assess the efficacy of assertiveness training has consisted either of inpatients in psychiatric facilities (Bornstein, Bellack, & Hersen, 1980), or of children and youth attending school (Filipczak, Archer, & Friedman, 1980; Fleming & Fleming, 1982). Table 1 illustrates the range of subject's character-

TABLE 1

STUDY:	BERLER et. al., 1982	BORNSTEIN et. al., 1977	BORNSTEIN et. al., 1980
SUBJECTS:	3 LD disabled boys	4 unassertive children	4 inpatient, aggressive childre

TARGET BEHAVIOR(S):	- eye contact
	- appro. verbal
	- request new
	  behavior
		- ratio; eye
		  contact,
		  special duration
		- loudness of speech
		- requests new
		  behavior
		- overall assertions
			- positive and
			  negative asserti
			- eye contact/
			  speech developme
			- hostile tone
			- request for new
			  behavior
			- overall assertio

MULTIPLE MEASURES:	no	yes	yes
ANALOG MEASUREMENT:	yes (12)	yes	yes (BAI-C)
GENERAL SCORES:	yes (8)	yes (3)	no
GENERAL EFFECTS:	yes, moderate	yes	--
GENERAL TRAINER RESPONDENT:	yes	not specified (multiple trainers used)	not specified (multiple trainers used)
GENERAL EFFECT:	yes	--	--
TRAINING STRATEGY:	behavior Model	behavioral Model	behavior Model
DIRECT MEASURE:	yes	no	no
FOLLOW UP:	1 month (effects)	2 & 4 weeks (effects)	1-26 weeks, (incompleted effects across Ss and behaviors)
COLLATERAL MESURES:	yes	no	no
COMPARATIVE ANALYSIS:	yes	no	no
REINFORCEMENT IN NATIONAL ENVIRONMENT:	yes	no	no
SOCIALLY VALIDATED EFFECT:	yes	no	no

TABLE 1 (continued)

	FLEMING & FLEMING 1980	GLEBINK et. al., 1968	LOCHMAN et. al., 1984
SUBJECTS:	48 EMR children	6 emotionally disturbed boys	76 appresive boys
TARGET BEHAVIOR(S):	assertion	verbal responses to 14 situation(s) (frustration questionnaire)	no specific target target behaviors mentioned
MULTIPLE MEASURES:	no	no	yes
ANALOGY MEASUREMENT:	yes (6)	yes (4)	not specific
GENERAL SCORES:	yes (4)	yes (4)	no
GENERAL EFFECTS:	yes	no	--
GENERAL TRAINER RESPONDENT:	not specified	no	no
GENERAL EFFECT:	--	--	--
TRAINING STRATEGY:	structured learning plus other procedures	game format	not specific
DIRECT MEASURE:	yes	yes	yes
FOLLOW-UP:	--	no	1 month effect
COLLATERAL MEASURES:	--	no	yes
COMPARATIVE ANALYSIS:	--	no	yes
REINFORCEMENT IN NATURAL ENVIRONMENT:	--	no	no
SOCIALLY VALIDATED EFFECT:	--	no	no

TABLE 1 (continued)

	MATSON et. al., 1980	MEREDITH et. al., 1980	MICHELSON et. al., 1980
SUBJECTS:	2 emotionally disturbed moderately retarded boys	20 mildly retarded young adults	61 boys socially maladjusted
TARGET BEHAVIORS:	- physical gestures - facial manners - eye contact - number of words spoken - voice intonation - overall social skill	- positive responses - negative responses	- smiles - app. reg. - regard - appreciation
MULTIPLE MEASURES:	yes	no	yes
ANALOGY MEASUREMENT:	yes (5)	yes (6)	not specific
GENERAL SCORES:	yes (5)	no	no
GENERAL EFFECTS:	yes	--	--
GENERAL TRAINER RESPONDENT:	no	no	no
GENERAL EFFECT:	--	--	--
TRAINING STRATEGY:	behavioral format	response shaping and guidelines	behavioral format plus role reversal and homework
DIRECT MEASURE:	no	no	yes
FOLLOW-UP:	4-6 weeks (effects)	No	1 year
COLLATERAL MEASURES:	no	no	yes
COMPARATIVE ANALYSIS:	no	yes	yes
REINFORCEMENT IN NATURAL ENVIRONMENT:	no	no	no
SOCIALLY VALIDATED EFFECT:	yes	no	no

istics in the studies reviewed. The availability of professional staff in inpatient facilities, combined with the need for such skills in the clients, makes this setting a prime target for research in assertion training. Its use with children and youth in outpatient settings requires increased efforts in testing the efficacy of assertion training. Schools, day care settings, and outpatient medical facilities offer the possibility of this treatment being tested with target subjects in these settings.

The subjects of the studies reviewed have been diagnosed as emotionally disturbed children (Giebink, Stover, & Fahl, 1968); learning disabled children (Berler, Gross, & Drabman, 1982); aggressive children (Lochman, Burch, Curry, & Lampron, 1984); unassertive children (Bornstein, Bellack, & Hersen, 1977); and mentally retarded children (Fleming & Fleming, 1982; Meredith, Saxon, Doleys, & Kyzer, 1980). More research is needed with these clinical populations, particularly emotionally disturbed, severely emotionally disturbed, and learning disabled children. Additionally, other clinical groups in which assertion training needs to be initially tested are moderately retarded individuals and socially withdrawn children.

Observable Components of Assertion

Table 1 also illustrates the range of behaviors that have been targeted for training. There are several common, observable behaviors that have been trained as components of assertion across a number of studies. Eye contact (Berler et al., 1982; Bornstein et al., 1977; Bornstein et al., 1980; Matson et al., 1980); request for new behavior (Berler et al., 1982; Bornstein et al., 1977; Bornstein et al., 1980; Michelson, Mannarino, Marchione, Stern, Figueroa, & Beck, 1983); and verbal content (Matson, Kazdin, & Esveldt-Dawson, 1980; Berler et al., 1982) are common target behaviors in assertion training studies.

Some research studies did not measure or target specific behaviors, but rather attempted to train a wide range of positive verbal responses while extinguishing negative behaviors (Giebink et al., 1968; Meredith et al., 1980). From a behavioral perspective, it is more efficient for assessment and training purposes to pinpoint specific observable components of assertion. By pinpointing the specific components of assertion, the trainer can precisely determine which components need to be trained to higher levels of occurrence.

Observable components are usually quantified either as occurring or not occurring (Matson et al., 1980). However with some behaviors, the frequency of occurrence is an important measure (e.g., the number of requests for new behavior) and, therefore, necessary. Other behaviors (voice intonation, loudness of speech and a global assessment of overall assertion) appear to be best measured with a Likert-type rating scale.

Multiple Measures

Table 1 provides two columns regarding measurement issues. The next column (see Table 1) indicates whether multiple measures of assertion were taken. Multiple measures were recorded if the researcher collected more than one type of data (e.g., collecting data on both observable behaviors and on a subjective rating system). It is advisable to include a subjective measure of overall assertion in combination with the assessment of observable components to provide a standard by which to judge the clinical significance of the treatment effect (Kazdin, 1977; Wolf, 1978). Training progress that produces changes in global subjective ratings that are concurrent with changes in observable behavior socially validate the objective quantitative measures as being crucial determinants of qualitative change. Social validation data have been collected in social skills research (Bornstein et al., 1977; Matson et al., 1980). This methodology should be continued as researchers investigate new sets of target behaviors.

For the practicing clinician, it might be more beneficial to utilize the normative comparison method in selecting observable components of assertion (Goldsmith & McFall, 1975). An analysis of peers judged to be assertive in target situations can identify the specific behaviors that should be targeted.

In everyday practice, there are three common measurements used to assess assertion: behavioral observations, peer sociometric rating scales, and teacher ratings (Gresham, 1981). Global ratings, in contrast to direct observational data by either teachers or peers are the most cost-effective, and can be used for large-scale screening (Hops, 1983). Rating systems being somewhat insensitive to treatment effects, can be useful as an initial screening device, if found to be reliable over time (Greenwood, Walker, & Hops, 1970). There are several commercially available screening assessment instruments. For example, the Social Assessment Manual for Preschool Level (SAMPLE) measures the child's rate of social interaction and contact through naturalistic observation, child's adeptness through teacher ratings and sociometric ratings from peers (Greenwood, Todd, & Walker, 1978).

Analog Measurement

Analog measurement (via role-playing) is used to train deficient skills to criterion in a relatively short period of time. It is usually not feasible to train assertion in the natural environment, in large part due to the relative infrequency of situations requiring assertion. Therefore, measurement and training of skills in a contrived environment is a more practical approach. However, as the next several sections of this paper indicate, it is necessary to eventually measure the behavior in the natural environment(s) and insure that its occurrence obtains reinforcement.

In most studies, researchers utilized a set number of role-playing scenes to teach the subject to acquire the component behaviors involved in assertion. The number of role-playing training scenes used (in parentheses in Table 2) can be from as few as four (Giebink et al., 1968) or can be comprised of an entire set of individualized role-playing scenes (e.g., the Behavioral Assertiveness Test for Children, Bornstein et al., 1980). Some role-playing scenes are designed to measure positive assertion (Bornstein et al., 1980) such as giving compliments (Matson et al., 1980); initiating conversation (Meredith et al., 1980); and asking for help (Matson et al., 1980). Negative assertion can be trained in scenes which present situations requiring requests and appropriate responses to negative statements (Matson et al., 1980).

The measurement of social skills in research laboratory conditions has generally been conducted in a standardized manner (i.e., the scene is role-played, the subject's response is recorded, no feedback is given during the assessment of skills). Results have been shown to vary if assessment conditions produce reinforcement for appropriate responding, in both "normal" and inpatient children (Kazdin, Matson, & Esveldt-Dawson, 1981). Therefore, data collected in assessments conducted without differential reinforcement contingencies may be an underestimate of capability. The role of motivation (i.e., reinforcement contingencies) needs to be considered in the assessment of assertion in analog measurement.

Assessing Generalization Across Untrained Scenes

The measurement of assertive behavior before and after training in novel role-playing scenes provides data which identifies the extent to which generalized behavior change has occurred to a range of interpersonal situations. This is assessed by having training occur only on selected scenes. Assessment is then conducted on nontrained or novel scenes to evaluate the generality of the treatment effect. Since only a small sample of scenes can be used in training, this is an important measure. Table 1 indicates that the majority of the studies have assessed generalization to novel situations.

When data are collected generalization has been readily obtained to untrained scenes (Berler et al., 1982; Bornstein et al., 1977; Fleming & Fleming, 1982; Matson et al., 1980). Bornstein et al. (1977) obtained effects to untrained scenes in both post-training assessment and follow-up assessments. Assessing for generalization across untrained scenes is as important for research interests as it is for the practitioner treating clients. One cannot assume that the sample of scenes used for training constitutes the range of conditions requiring assertion. Therefore, measurement of behavior in untrained scenes is vital in therapy to estimate the generality of assertion skills after training. Therapists should periodically check for generalization during the course of therapy to insure that therapy is producing a generalized set of acquired skills.

Assessing Generalization Across Novel Trainers

Unless there are data to suggest otherwise, it is possible that the sole employment of one or a few trainers may produce assertion under restricted conditions (i.e., only with the person(s) used in the training). This is a realistic concern in many therapy situations where only one therapist is used. Generally, the ultimate criterion for judging the effectiveness of the training is for the target child or youth to exhibit assertive behavior to his or her peers under the right conditions. Researchers and therapists should make provisions to measure the subject's capability of responding to novel respondents (peer and/or adult, if relevant).

The research studies have attended less to generalization across novel trainers than to generalization across untrained scenes (see Table 1). In some cases, the research study failed to specify if novel trainers were used in the assessments despite indication that more than one trainer was used during training of each component skill (Bornstein et al., 1977). Generalization across novel people is just as crucial as generalization across novel scenes.

Training Strategy

Most of the research studies utilized a four-step behavioral model in training assertion: (a) instructions, (b) modeling, (c) behavioral rehearsal, and (d) feedback (Berler et al., 1982; Bornstein et al., 1977; Matson et al., 1980). This is indicated in Table 1 by specifying if a behavioral model was used.

In most cases, as a result of utilizing a multiple baseline across behaviors design, the training program proceeded by teaching one specific behavior to criterion at a time. For example, Bornstein et al. (1980) initially trained four inpatient children to increase their rate of eye contact to total speech duration. Upon reaching an acceptable duration of eye contact, the children were then trained to reduce their hostile tone. With both eye contact and hostile tone at specified levels, the children were then taught the skill of requesting a new behavior. This procedure resulted in efficient acquisition of acceptable levels of all three target behaviors.

Curriculum materials that teach assertion and other social skills are available. The Preparation Through Responsive Educational Programming (PREP) is a comprehensive program that teaches a variety of social assertion skills in a curriculum materials format (Filipczak et al., 1980). Another comprehensive program (Procedures for Establishing Effective Relationship Skills or PEERS) is designed to facilitate the development of social skills in socially withdrawn handicapped children (Hops, Fleischman, Guild, Paine, Wahler, & Greenwood, 1978). A similarly designed program for negative/aggressive children (Reprogramming Environmental Contingencies for Effective Social Skills or RECESS) has been field tested with encouraging results (Walker, Street, Garrett, Hops, Crossen, & Greenwood, 1978).

Assessing Behavior in Its Natural Context (Direct Measure)

It has been suggested that role-playing data may not approximate direct measures of behavior (Bellack, Hersen, & Lamparski, 1979; McNamara & Blumer, 1982). For example, in a study with 58 elementary school children, data on social competence in role-playing situations did not significantly correlate with either peer or teacher ratings of child behavior (Matson, Esveldt-Dawson, & Kazdin, 1983). Low correlations between role-play measures and criterion (direct observation, sociometric, and teacher ratings) measures have been replicated (Van Hasselt, Hersen, & Bellack, 1981). Van Hasselt et al. (1981) found a low test-retest reliability of role-playing measures. Despite some limitations in those studies (e.g., subjects in the samples were not "problematic"), this data cannot be overlooked. Research with adult psychiatric clinical populations substantiates further the possibility that analog data may be an invalid predictor of treatment outcome (Bellack, Hersen, & Turner, 1979). Therefore, measuring treatment effects in the natural context would be as much a practical concern as it is a research concern.

Recent applied research has begun to collect direct measures of social competence in addition to role-playing measures (see Table 1). For example, in testing the efficacy of structured learning therapy, a direct measure was taken immediately following and one week after training (Fleming & Fleming, 1982). Two situations were set up in the natural environment to test the child's social assertion skills. In one situation, a confederate child attempted to push ahead of the subject. In a second situation, a game format was used to test the child's negative assertion skills when attacked verbally by a confederate child during the game. Unfortunately, generalization of the treatment effect was not realized to this direct measure.

Other research has resulted in similar findings regarding lack of generalization to more natural contexts (Berler et al., 1982; Bornstein et al., 1980). One study found some generalization to the classroom and home situation (Lochman, Burch, Curry, & Lampron, 1984). For the most part, research studies have either failed to collect direct measures of assertive behavior or have failed to obtain such when measured. The technology of generalization is in an infancy stage in the area of social assertion training. To begin understanding what variables may be responsible for generalization, current and future research studies should measure variables operating in the social ecology of the natural setting. This is as important for the researcher as it is for the clinician. Clinicians must collect data on assertion in the natural environment. Data collection by trained peers, in simulated situations, is one possibility of gathering such data.

Follow-up Assessment

In addition to a direct measure of social assertion, it is also important to assess the durability of the treatment effect. Follow-up data collected on role-playing scenes and/or direct measures of the behavior indicates the degree to which the behavior maintains after treatment. More research studies are needed which assess maintenance of skill after termination of therapy (Jackson, King, & Heller, 1981).

In general, studies that have collected follow-up data over a period of two to six weeks past therapy have found durable effects (Berler et al., 1982; Lochman et al., 1984; Matson et al., 1980). However, in a longer follow-up period (4 to 26 weeks), durability of treatment effects was found to be inconsistent across subjects and behaviors (Bornstein et al., 1980). In particular, Bornstein et al. (1980) found requests for new behavior particularly resistent to long-term maintenance for two of the subjects.

Future research studies need to address the issue of durability and begin to develop methods that can increase the probability of obtaining long-term gains. For the practitioner in the field it is particularly important. Gains made in therapy that do not maintain over time, do little to improve the subject's capability in dealing with future interpersonal situations that require assertion. Follow-up in clinical practice should be conducted over the long-term, with "booster" sessions provided if needed.

Assessing Collateral Measures

As is evident from Table 1, few studies assess the possibility of side effects to collateral behaviors. Yet, one measure of the breadth of the treatment program would be generalization across different, untreated, behaviors. Teaching children or youth to assert themselves in situations where it is required should have the effect of reducing inappropriate behaviors that were functioning previously adaptive in those situations. In studies that treated aggressive children, a good measure of the efficacy of the treatment would have been a measure of the incidence of their aggression in these situations.

In treating learning disabled children, Berler et al. (1982) found that duration of speech increased slightly after verbal content was trained. Increasing this behavior could improve a child's ability to interact successfully with his/her peers. Duration of speech would seem to be a variable that would promote a persistent assertive response. In a second example of assessing collateral behaviors, independent play and adaptive and maladaptive peer interactions were measured while assertive behavior was trained (Michelson et al., 1983).

It is commonly assumed that changing the child's ability to assert himself or herself in interpersonal situations will decrease behaviors that are less desirable. However, this may not be the case. Future research studies need to address the possibility of positive side effects.

Conducting a Comparative Analysis

Minimally, in a development of a behavioral technology, a body of research should be available that tests the efficacy of a package treatment strategy against a control condition. Skills training is an entire set of procedures. In most studies addressing this comparison, skills training has proved to be substantially better than conditions usually serving as attention only or interact controls (e.g.,

Berler et al., 1982; Fleming & Fleming, 1982; Lochman et al., 1984; Meredith et al., 1980). In a study comparing a more powerful treatment condition with social skills training, several measures showed significant differences at a one-year follow-up for the social skills training group only (Michelsen et al., 1983). Neither the interpersonal problem solving training group or the control group maintained gains in post-training assessment of assertion. As the technology develops, comparisons with other treatment modalities (psychotherapy, medication, etc.) need to be conducted. It is initially important to identify if a given treatment works. But the next question then becomes, does it work better than already existing models? The results of comparative research constitute the most compelling resources for practitioners to treat a referred problem in a certain therapeutic manner.

Assessing Reinforcement Contingencies in the Natural Context

The maintenance of the behavior in the natural environment, and the extinction of undesirable problematic behaviors, rests on the ability of the natural environment to reinforce the occurrence of that behavior. This measure has not been assessed in any of the studies reviewed. Stokes and Baer (1977) indicate that the occurrence of an acquired behavior needs to be viewed in terms of recruiting the communities of natural (peer) reinforcement. Research has not begun to address this variable (i.e., measuring the rate of reinforcement for newly acquired skills). Identifying the social, ecological conditions needed to support a behavior may provide answers to how one can best obtain generalization to untrained stimuli, other trainers and maintenance in the natural context. Reinforcement from peers and parents for assertive behavior will increase the likelihood for maintenance (Jackson, King, & Heller, 1981).

Social Validation of Treatment Effects

The use of social validation techniques as a method of documenting the quality of quantitative changes was discussed earlier and is presented in detail elsewhere (Kazdin, 1977; Wolf, 1978). The additional concern in measuring the quality of the newly acquired social assertive behavior is that the criterion group selected as nonproblematic should be a truly representative group. Sex and age are important factors in selecting a representative nonproblematic peer group, given the rapid changes that occur in social behavior with young children (Hops et al., 1978).

An example of the validation of the treatment effect was the methodology used in the Matson et al. (1980) study. In determining if the rates of the target behaviors after training were at a competent level, four nonproblematic children were assessed in the targeted interpersonal situations. The results indicated that post training data of the target subjects were above the normative levels of nonproblematic children. The practical implication of this is obviously that training was effective in changing the level of positive interpersonal skills to a significant level.

INTERVIEWING SKILLS

Interviewing skills are crucial in obtaining employment. The training of acceptable interviewing behavior has recently been addressed in the behavioral literature.

A comprehensive program was developed by Azrin and his colleagues in addressing a number of skills needed to obtain employment (Azrin, Flores, & Kaplan, 1975). The Job-Finding Club was a training program that taught a number of skills to a group of subjects who fulfilled the criteria of being unemployed. In a comparison with a control condition, Job-Finding Club subjects were able to obtain more jobs, make more money, be more satisfied with their jobs and keep them longer than the control subjects.

The most comprehensive study of training interviewing skills analyzed 12 separate behaviors with 36 youths (25% had committed juvenile offenses) in a federally funded program (Heimburg, Cunningham, Stankey, & Blankenberg, 1982). Training consisted of role-playing an interview based on descriptions of two positions. The positions selected for the role-playing scenario were positions for which most of the subjects were qualified. Training sessions were for 90 minutes, twice weekly. Each of the behaviors was taught to criterion prior to the training of the next targeted behavior.

Data were collected via an actual interview with a number of public and industry employers rating each subject's performance. Two groups of social skills training (two and four sessions of skill training) were compared with two control groups (discussion only and delayed treatment). Employers indicated that subjects from the two experimental groups were consistently rated as sufficiently competent in the interview to consider for employment based on the presented videotaped interview.

Two other research studies dealt with training interview skills to mildly retarded males (Kelly, Wildman, & Berber, 1980) and females (Hall, Sheldon-Wildgen, & Sherman, 1980). Kelly et al. (1980) trained four specific behaviors in improving interview skills: (a) provide favorable information about their previous work experience, (b) offer positive information about oneself, (c) ask questions of the interviewer regarding the job, and (d) express verbal interest and enthusiasm. Ten standard interview questions were developed to train these skills. The interview questions were socially validated by surveying several personnel managers on commonly utilized interview questions. In addition to the assessment of each of these behaviors across a multiple baseline, pre- and post-measures of an interview conducted by two novel managers served as a direct measure of interviewing behavior.

All four subjects increased the frequency of targeted behaviors as a function of training. Subjects showed gains from baseline measures in all five areas rated by other managers naive to the purpose of the research. Managers rated the subjects significantly higher in: (a) apparent interest in working, (b) competence and ability, (c) likelihood of being hired, (d) having a well rounded personality, and (e) work and training experience.

A second study conducted in the subjects' group home trained three areas comprising interview skills: (a) office skills, (b) interview skills, and (c) application skills (Hall et al., 1980). Office skills included introducing oneself to the receptionist, stating the purpose for being there and following directions. Interview skills involved the presence of good posture, appropriate voice tone and rate, and asking and answering questions appropriately. Application skills involved written responses to standard job application questions. During the training of this latter skill, 15 forms were used. A different from was used in assessing for generalization.

To measure the generality of the training, a probe procedure was instituted after the training of each skill area to assess performance. These probes were held in a downtown office with three novel receptionists used in each probe. All target skills were measured during this probe. A special probe at the end of all training was conducted in a new office complex, with different application forms and different interviewers. The subjects improved in all skill areas as a function of training during regular probes. Special probe data indicated generalization of skills for office and application areas, but a decrease for interviewing skills (for two subjects).

There is a need for increased research efforts in this area. The current trend is to train handicapped people earlier in their school career on functional vocational activities (Trach & Rusch, in press). Testing of behavioral training strategies with different types of handicapped children and youth are needed. Generalization across trainers, stimuli and settings needs to be assessed. The research available has ingeniously succeeded in collecting a direct measure of interview behavior through simulations in novel offices that closely approximate "real-life" conditions. The use of surveys assessing potential manager's evaluation of subject's interview behavior provides a nice validation of the training program and the obtained results. Increased attention to follow-up measures as well as comparative studies is needed.

CONVERSATIONAL SKILLS

Subjects and Setting

A majority of the studies received have focused on the training of conversational skills with mentally retarded adolescents (Kelly, Furman, Phillips, Hathorn, & Wilson, 1979; Tofte-Tipps, Mendonca, & Peach, 1982). The initial study giving the impetus to investigate conversational skills training targeted four delinquent females (Minkin, Braukmann, Minkin, Timbers, Timbers, Fixsen, Phillips, & Wolfe, 1976).

The efficacy and feasibility of conducting conversational skills training with other types of children and youth who are deficient in their ability to converse successfully with peers and/or adults needs to be studied. Table 2 reveals that all but one study has dealt with developmentally disabled children. Its use with socially withdrawn children, emotionally disturbed children, and other types of handicapped children and youth is needed. The inability to initiate and maintain a conversation can affect the individual's ability to socialize with his or her peer group. Friendships, appearing likeable, and "fitting in" can be positively affected by increased conversational ability (Bradlyn, Himadi, Crimmins, Christoff, Graves, & Kelly, 1983).

Assessing Observable Components of Conversational Ability

The target behaviors measured as observable components of conversational ability are given in Table 2. Minkin and colleagues (1976) socially validated three components of conversational ability by identifying observable behaviors that differentiated good versus poor conversants as judged by raters. The number of short, positive feedback statements made when someone else was talking, the number of conversational questions asked, and the time spent talking were three behaviors that occurred frequently in good conversants. Eye contact was measured in several studies (Cipani, 1980; Tofte-Tipps et al., 1982). Kelly, Furman, Phillips, Hathorn, and Wilson (1979) measured informational facts and invitations to engage in an activity in addition to frequency of questions in assessing conversational ability of two retarded adolescent males.

Either frequency or interval recording systems have been used to measure most target behaviors. In addition, several research studies have utilized ratings of overall conversational ability to validate the observable targets of the intervention (Bradlyn et al., 1983; Cipani, 1980; Minkin et al., 1976).

Analog Measurement

Table 2 indicates that the majority of the studies have utilized conversational role-playing as the method of assessing ability (Kelly, Wildman, Urey, & Thurman, 1979; Tofte-Tipps et al., 1982). In most cases, the subject is instructed to engage the other

TABLE 2

STUDY:	BRADLYN et. al., 1982	CIPANI 1980	KELLY, WILDMAN, UREY & THURMAN, 1979
SUBJECTS/ SETTINGS:	5 MR adolescents	Emotional disturbed adolescents	10 MR adolescent behavior problems
TARGET BEHAVIOR(S):	- conv. quest. - self disclosure statement - acknowledge comments	- conv. quest - positive feedback	- questions - self disclosure statement - complimenting comments
ANALOG MEASUREMENT:	yes (8 min)	yes (4 min)	yes (4 min)
GENERAL CONVERSANTS:	yes	no	no
EFFECTS:	yes	--	--
TRAINING STRATEGY:	behavioral format	behavioral format	behavioral format
DIRECT MEASURE:	no	no	no
FOLLOW-UP:	5 mo. (effects)	No	1 mo. (effects)
COLLATERAL MEASURE:	no	yes	no
COMPARATIVE ANALOG:	no	no	no
ENVIRONMENT:	no	no	no
SOCIAL VALIDATED EFFECTS:	yes	yes	no

	KELLY, FURMAN, PHILLIPS, HATHORN and WILSON, 1979	TOFFLE-TIPPS, et. al., 1982
SUBJECTS/ SETTING:	2 MR adolescent males	2 developmentally adolescents
TARGET BEHAVIOR(S):	- inform facts - questions - invitations to engage in activity	10 target behaviors

TABLE 2 (continued)

	KELLY, FURMAN, PHILLIPS, HATHORN and WILSON, 1979	TOFFLE-TIPPS, et. al., 1982
ANALOG MEASUREMENT:	yes (structured questions)	yes (1 minute)
GENERAL CONVERSANTS:	yes	yes
EFFECTS:	yes	adults (yes) peers; no
TRAINING STRATEGY:	behavioral format	behavioral format
DIRECT MEASURE:	yes, 20 minute free play (effects)	no
FOLLOW-UP:	3 weeks (effect)	1 month (effects)
COLLATERAL MEASURE:	yes	no
COMPARATIVE ANALOG:	yes	no
ENVIRONMENT:	no	no
SOCIAL VALIDATED EFFECTS:	no	no

conversant in conversation for a period of time, without any suggestion as to topic. The length of the role-play can be from one-minute (Tofte-Tipps et al., 1982) to eight minutes (Kelly, Furman, Phillips, Hathorn, & Wilson, 1979). Usually, the confederates are instructed as to how many times they can initiate conversation, or the number of questions they can ask.

Kelly, Furman, Phillips, Hathorn, and Wilson (1979), utilized a different format in having the role-respondent present 13 structured sentences involving questions, compliments, and self-descriptions. The subject's response to each of these statements was then measured. Possibly, future research studies could measure the subjects' responses to structured statements as well as in extemporaneous conversations. Measuring conversation under different lengths is also needed to determine the generality of effects. Finally, the ability of the subject to adequately change the topic of conversation (when they may be unfamiliar with topic) needs to be addressed.

Generalization Across Novel Conversants

Similar to the training of assertion and interviewing skills, training conversational skills often occurs with one therapist. Do the results obtained with the therapist represent how the client would perform with other people? The majority of the studies has assessed and found generalization occurring to novel conversants (Minkin et al., 1976; Kelly, Wildman, Urey, & Thurman, 1979). An interesting finding in one study was that generalization was obtained to novel adults but not same-aged children (Tofte-Tipps et al., 1982).

Future research needs to examine generalization across conversants that are representative of peers found in the child's natural environments. Generalization of conversational ability is important for the same reasons as cited in the assertive literature review for the practicing clinician.

Training Strategy

The training strategy has generally included the following four components: instructions, modeling, behavioral rehearsal, and feedback after rehearsal. In several studies, trainers used a group-instruction format (Minkin et al., 1976; Kelly, Wildman, Urey, & Thurman, 1979). One potential problem with group training can be increased variably in the treatment effect, due to lack of individual instruction. Kelly, Wildman, Urey, and Thurman (1979) found variability in the effect, but the levels of all targeted behaviors were above baseline. This problem can be remediated in practice by providing one-to-one training sessions with subjects who do not reach criterion on each targeted behavior. Future research needs to address the treatment effectiveness and efficiency of group strategies versus one-on-one sessions.

Direct Measure and Follow-up

Obviously, a direct measure is as important here as with the two previous skills reviewed. As Table 2 indicates, only one study measured the effects of conversational skills training on conversation in the natural context (Kelly, Furman, Phillips, Hathorn, & Wilson, 1979). In this study, researchers collected data during several 20-minute observations on the amount of talk, play, and lack of interaction during free-play at one and two weeks following. Both adolescents showed gains in free-play social interaction in both follow-up assessments and decreases in the amount of time that was void of interaction. In the same study, follow-up data on role-playing scenes indicated some loss of question asking behavior in both subjects.

Maintenance data has been obtained in some studies. Researchers conducting follow-ups found treatment to be durable (Bradlyn et al., 1983; Kelly, Furman, Phillips, Hathorn, & Wilson, 1979; Kelly, Wildman, Urey, & Thurman, 1979). Future research needs to continue to address direct measures of conversation in the natural environment, perhaps validated by peer sociometric ratings. Additionally, continuing to measure the durability of the treatment effect in follow-up assessments is also needed.

Collateral Measures and Comparative Analyses

As Table 2 indicates, the majority of the research has failed either to measure collateral behavior or to provide comparisons between different treatment techniques. Both of these are crucial to the development of a technology for training conversational ability. Cipani (1980) anecdotally reported a positive side effect of conversational skills training. The subject, who had never been on an interview, was scheduled for an interview after training and successfully landed a position. Kelly, Furman, Phillips, Hathorn, and Wilson (1979) also found collateral changes in subjects' rates of play (collateral measure) and talk with others during measurement of behavior during free-play.

Future research should investigate the positive side effects of training conversational skills. Possible collateral measures might be aggression, play behavior, compliance, disruptive behavior, social and/or dating behaviors toward members of the opposite sex, and other areas of social competence. Comparative analyses in future research might include contrasts of skill training with discussion only, traditional psychotherapy methods and contingency management procedures.

Reinforcement Contingencies in the Natural Environment

Research has been lacking in measuring the rate of peer reinforcement for the newly acquired skill in the natural context (see Table 2). Future research needs to increase the measurement of conversation in the natural context, and to measure the response of the social environment to such behavior.

Social Validation of Treatment Effect

How much is enough? This question can be assessed by collecting subjective global measures before and after training, rating the degree of change. Table 2 presents the findings of this review on studies collecting this data. The general methodology is to collect videotape segments during baseline and post-training and present them randomly to raters who are asked to rate the degree of conversational ability (Bradlyn et al., 1983). Minkin et al. (1976) utilized subjective ratings of university female students rated as good conversants as the training standard for the female subjects of the study. Average training ratings of the subjects was 4.3 (one to seven scale). This average rating surpassed the rating of their peers in a sample of junior high school female students (3.7) and closely approximated the mean rating (5.0) of the university students. This data enhances the credibility of the treatment effect obtained. Cipani (1980) utilized data collected on global ratings on a number of dimensions to indicate the strength of the treatment effect.

Social validation data should be collected to insure that the results in conversational ability are clinically significant (i.e., noticeable to people and thus probably reflect a qualitative as well as a quantitative change, [Wolf, 1978]).

SUMMARY

Much has developed in the field's understanding of treating behavioral deficits in areas of social competence in handicapped children and adolescents. Researchers have amassed a body of literature studying this area, but more needs to be done. Clinicians have a set of tools to begin treating such problems. There is a valid and useful methodology for measuring specific behaviors that comprise competence in each of the three areas reviewed in this paper. Furthermore, the research has clearly identified that, by using a behavioral training format, these skills can be taught.

Generalization has been a more complex issue in identifying a technology for obtaining results. While it does appear that it can be obtained, it is not clear under what conditions it becomes a more probable occurrence. Further efforts to identify the conditions of the social ecology of newly acquired skills and its reinforcement (or lack thereof) are needed. Methods aimed at manipulating such conditions may prove fruitful in facilitating generalization across relevant settings, time, other stimuli, and behaviors.

REFERENCES

Azrin, N. H., Flores, T., & Kaplan, S. J. (1975). Job-finding club: A group assisted program for obtaining employment. *Behavior Research and Therapy*, 13, 17-27.

Ballard, M., Corman, L., Gottlieb, J., & Kaufman, M. L. (1977). Improving the social status of mainstreamed retarded children. *Journal of Educational Psychology*, 69, 605-611.

Bellack, A. S., Hersen, M., & Turner, S. M. (1979). Relationship of role playing and knowledge of appropriate behavior to assertion in the natural environment. *Journal of Consulting and Clinical Psychology*, 47, 670-678.

Bellack, A. S., Hersen, M., & Lamparski, D. (1979). Role-play tests for assessing social skills: Are they valid? Are they useful? *Journal of Consulting and Clinical Psychology*, 47, 335-342.

Berler, E. S., Gross, A. M., & Drabman, R. S. (1982). Social skills training with children: Proceed with caution. *Journal of Applied Behavior Analysis*, 15, 41-153.

Bornstein, M. R., Bellack, A. S., & Hersen, M. (1977). Social skills training for unassertive children: A multiple baseline analysis. *Journal of Applied Behavior Analysis*, 10, 183-195.

Bornstein, M., Bellack, A. S., & Hersen, J. (1980). Social skills training for highly aggressive children: Treatment in an inpatient psychiatric setting. *Behavior Modification*, 4, 173-186.

Bradlyn, A. S., Himadi, W. G., Crimmins, D. B., Christoff, K. A., Graves, K. G., & Kelly, J. A. (1983). Conversational skills training for retarded adolescents. *Behavior Therapy*, 14, 314-325.

Charles, D. C. & McGrath, K. (1962). The relationship of peer and staff ratings to release from institutionalization. *American Journal of Mental Deficiency*, 67, 414-417.

Cipani, E. (1980). Measuring the utility of a reinforcer: The modification of academic and social behavior in an emotionally disturbed student. *Behavioral Engineering*, 6, 109-116.

Combs, M. L. & Slaby, D. A. (1977). Skills training with children. In B. Lahey & A. E. Kazdin's (Eds.), *Advances in Clinical Child Psychology: (Vol. 1)*, New York: Plenum.

Filipczak, J., Archer, M., & Friedman, R. B. (1980). In school social skills training: Use with disruptive adolescents. *Behavior Modification*, 4, 243-263.

Fleming, E. R. & Fleming, D. C. (1982). Social skill training for educable mentally retarded children. *Education and Training of the Mentally Retarded*, 17, 44-50.

Giebink, J. W., Stover, D. D., & Fahl, M. A. (1968). Teaching adaptive responses to frustration to emotionally disturbed boys. *Journal of Consulting and Clinical Psychology*, 32, 366-368.

Goldsmith, J. B. & McFall, R.M. (1975). Developmental evaluation of an interpersonal skill training program for psychiatric inpatient. *Journal of Abnormal Psychology*, 84, 51-52.

Gottlieb, J. (1975). Attitudes toward retarded children: Effects of labeling and behavioral-aggressiveness. *Journal of Educational Psychology*, 67, 581-585.

Gresham, F. M. (1981). Assessment of children's social skills. *Journal of School Psychology*, 19, 120-133.

Greenwood, C. R., Walker, H. M., & Hops, H. (1970). Issues in social interaction/assessment withdrawal. *Exceptional Children*, 43, 490-499.

Greenwood, C. R., Todd, N. M., & Walker, H. M. (1978). Social assessment manual for preschool level (SAMPLE). Eugene Center of Oregon for Research in the Behavioral Education of the Handicapped, University of Oregon, Eugene.

Hall, C., Sheldon-Wildgen, J., & Sherman, J. A. (1980). Teaching job interview skills to retarded clients. *Journal of Applied Behavior Analysis*, 13, 433-442.

Heimburg, R. G., Cunningham, J., Stankey, J., & Blankenberg, R. (1982). Preparing unemployed youth for job interviews: A controlled evaluation of social skills training. *Behavior Modification*, 6, 299-322.

Hops, H. (1983). Children's social competence and skills: Current research practices and future directions. *Behavior Therapy*, 14, 3-18.

Hops, H., Fleischman, D. H., Guild, J. J., Paine, S. C., Wahler, H. M., & Greenwood, C. R. (1978). PEERS (Program for socially withdrawn children). Center of Oregon for Research in the Behavioral Education of the Handicapped. Center on Human Development, University of Oregon, Eugene.

Jackson, H. J., King, M. J., & Heller, V. R. (1981). Social skills assessment and training for mentally retarded persons: A review of research. *Australian Journal of Developmental Disabilities*, 7, 113-123.

Kagan, J. & Moss, H. A. (1962). *Birth to maturity: A study in psychological development*. New York: John Wiley.

Kazdin, A. E. (1977). Assessing the clinical or applied importance of behavior change through social validation. *Behavior Modification*, 1, 427-452.

Kazdin, A. E., Matson, J. L., & Esveldt-Dawson, K. (1981). Social skill performance among normal and psychiatric inpatient children as a function of assessment conditions. *Behavior Research and Therapy*, 19, 145-152.

Kelly, J. A., Furman, W., Phillips, J., Hathorn, S., & Wilson, T. (1979). Teaching conversational skills to retarded adolescents. *Child Behavior Therapy*, 1, 85-97.

Kelly, J. A., Wildman, B. G., & Berber, E. S. (1980). Small group behavioral training to improve the job interview skills repertoire of mildly retarded adolescents. *Journal of Applied Behavior Analysis*, 13, 461-471.

Kelly, J. A., Wildman, B. G., Urey, J. R., & Thurman, C. (1979). Group skills training to increase the conversational repertoire of retarded adolescents. *Child Behavior Therapy*, 1, 323-336.

Lochman, J. E., Burch, P. R., Curry, J. F., & Lampron, L. B. (1984). Treatment and generalization effects of cognitive-behavioral and goal setting interventions with aggressive boys. *Journal of Consulting and Clinical Psychology*, 52, 915-916.

Matson, J. L., Esveldt-Dawson, K., & Kazdin, A. E. (1983). Validation of methods for assessing social skills in children. *Journal of Clinical Psychology*, 12, 174-180.

Matson, J. L., Kazdin, A. E., & Esveldt-Dawson, K. (1980). Training interpersonal skills among mentally retarded and socially dysfunctional children. *Behavior Research and Therapy*, 18, 419-427.

McNamara, J. R. & Blumer, C. A. (1982). Role playing to assess social competence: Ecological validity considerations. *Behavior Modification*, 6, 519-549.

Meredith, R. L., Saxon, S., Doleys, D. M., & Kyzer, B. (1980). Social skills training with mildly retarded young adults. *Journal of Clinical Psychology*, 36, 1000-1009.

Michelson, L., Mannarino, A. P., Marchione, R. E., Stern, M., Figueroa, J., & Beck, S. (1983). A comparative outcome study of behavioral social skills training, interpersonal problem solving and non-directive control treatments with child psychiatric outpatients. *Behavior Research and Therapy*, 21, 545-556.

Minkin, N., Braukmann, C. J., Minkin, B. L., Timbers, G. D., Timbers, B. J., Fixsen, D. L., Phillips, E. L., & Wolfe, M. M. (1976). The social validation and training of conversational skills. *Journal of Applied Behavior Analysis*, 127-139.

Roff, M., Seels, B., & Golden, B. (1972). Social adjustment and personality development in children. Minneapolis: University of Minnesota Press.

Stokes, T. F. & Baer, D. M. (1977). An implicit technology of generalization. *Journal of Applied Behavior Analysis*, 10, 349-367.

Tofte-Tipps, S., Mendonca, P., & Peach, R. V. (1982). Training and generalization of social skills: A study with two developmentally handicapped socially isolated children. *Behavior Modification*, 6, 45-71.

Van Hasselt, V. B., Hersen, M., Whitehall, M. B., & Bellack, A. S. (1979). Social skill assessment and training for children: An evaluative review. *Behavior Research and Therapy*, 17, 413-437.

Van Hasselt, V. B., Hersen, M., & Bellack, A. S. (1981). The validity of role play tests for assessing social skills in children. *Behavior Therapy*, 12, 202-216.

Walker, H. M., Street, A., Garrett, B., Hops, H., Crossen, J., & Greenwood, C. R. (1978). Reprogramming environmental contingencies for effective social skills (RECESS): Consultant manual. Center of Oregon for Research in the Behavioral Education of the Handicapped, University of Oregon, Eugene.

Wolf, M. M. (1978). Social validity: The case for subjective measurement or how applied behavior analysis is finding its heart. *Journal of Applied Behavior Analysis*, 11, 203-214.

Leisure and Recreation of Exceptional Children: Theory and Practice

Sherwood B. Chorost

ABSTRACT. Exceptional children are often deprived of experiences necessary to function adequately among normal peers. Various authors have cited research indicating the habilitative effects of successful play upon the emotional, social, and cognitive skill deficits of these children. Application of behavior technology to promote specific skills can assist children with mild, moderate, severe, and profound handicaps to become more accepted and acceptable. Theoretical bases and practical applications of therapeutic leisure and recreation programs are discussed. Examples show how such activities can be designed to create an environment to facilitate the educational treatment of handicapped students.

The developmental unfolding of the child is complicated by what Dewey (1956) identifies as two fundamental conflicts: the child vs. the curriculum, and individual nature vs. social culture. In a process which seeks to direct development, major problems occur in the selection, timing and persistence of appropriate stimuli which operate on the instincts and impulses of the child. The questions of what stimuli are needed and what experiences will produce desirable ends fall to adults who must try to prepare children for their place in society.

The discovery of psychological stages of growth reveals a map of how children order certain experiences, and how they connect

Sherwood Chorost is affiliated with The College of Staten Island, City University of New York. Address correspondence to Dr. Sherwood B. Chorost at 201 Avon Road, Westfield, NJ 07090.

151

events. Studies of how individuals learn (Gordon, 1962; Bandura, 1977) have added to our pedagogical approaches of curriculum design. Research on perceptual and physical maturation (Ausubel, 1958; Gordon, 1962; Bruininks, 1974) on the growth of awareness of self and others, has led to notions of critical periods (Erikson, 1963; Piaget, 1972; Spitz, 1972). Critical periods are of paramount importance in timing the educative process. Observations on the needs and stages of emotional and social growth have increased understanding of essential experiences to promote readiness for interaction. And yet, many children lack the personal trust, confidence, initiative, and readiness to transform their energy into pleasurable, useful, and efficient ends.

Something in the process has failed — the child, the curriculum, social culture, or the interaction of the three. Based on a variety of incidence studies of deviancy reported by Meyen (1982), we know that at least 20% of school-age children exhibit learning and behavioral characteristics which significantly interfere with their educational process and personal-social development. The time-honored process of placing a child into a group of his peers for a portion of the day, and of presenting a series of tasks (curricula) to stimulate his ability to differentiate, integrate, and organize experience, often does *not* lead to success. Without success, the child's ego cannot or does not unfold. It does not produce the stage-linked achievements which society expects, and which leads to the ability to work and to play and to perpetuate the social system.

Experiences found to be sufficient to mold the raw material brought to the process by *most* children may not be sufficient to educate the handicapped child. For handicapped children, i.e., children with mental retardation, learning disability, emotional disorder, behavior disorder, etc., the basic education system often needs to be modified. The positive peer attitudes and behaviors so crucial for the development of effective growth patterns are frequently distorted for the handicapped child (Guralnick, 1978; Semmel & Chaney, 1979; Bartel & Guskin, 1980; Hewett & Forness, 1984). The social milieu is often experienced as negative or as severely restricted due to the isolative effects produced by protective parents, exclusionary social practices, and/or by the withdrawal patterns of the handicapped children themselves.

Throughout life, each person must deal with challenges to, and frustrations in, social-psychological growth. These challenges may be divided into four basic domains represented by specific developmental tasks progressing from infancy into adulthood. These domains are: *LOVE* (attachment and separation), *LANGUAGE* (understanding and communicating), *WORK* (skill acquisition and application), and *PLAY* (tension release and mastery). The roles of play, recreation and leisure will be discussed as they relate to the lives of handicapped children.

EFFECTS OF EARLY PLAY DEPRIVATION

Handicapped youngsters must often deal with unique impediments in their abilities to generate positive reinforcement from the environment. Some of these impediments may, of course, be based on genetic or biological factors. However, it is essentially the *effect* of limited positive mutual interaction in play which places them in a "high risk" category. Piaget (1972) and Murphy (1972) described the prototype of play, i.e., interaction and feedback, as occurring in the earliest stages of the parent-child relationship. After about six weeks of age, cognitive skills and reality testing undergo rapid growth and the child begins to sense a linkage with significant others. When early experiences of play do not lead to release of tension and to a sense of mastery over one's social surroundings, the stage is set for ominous patterns of withdrawal and depression. Without adequate images of successful play and a repertoire of play skills needed to engage in and sustain effective interaction, normalization of one's childhood is threatened. Deprivation in the area of play thus results in cognitive, emotional and/or social disabilities. By evaluating and understanding how a child fails to deal with the developmental tasks associated with the playing domain (leisure and recreation skills), adults may help him minimize his handicap. Strain (1982) stated that a

> plea for stimulation of play is no luxury. . . . We are convinced that play behavior, particularly in the young child, greatly influences nearly all facets of development. Not only can play help in working with children who are disturbed, but it is extremely important in preventing learning problems. (p. 160)

Rules and rituals emerge early in play activity in the form of spontaneous improvisations with materials, toys, and games (Spitz, 1972). In normal circumstances, encouragement by parents, family, teaching adults, and peers assists in reducing ambiguities and in promoting mutual affective bonding. Erikson stressed the powerful role of ritualized reassurance in play, and cited the deleterious effect of an inability to sublimate and bond through play.

Erikson (1963) observed that the "thing-world of play" (the microsphere) had its own rules (p. 221). In his studies of play constructions of normal four- and five-year olds from different backgrounds, blocks and toys were offered to children with a request to build something and to tell a story about it (Erikson, 1972). A striking feature of this research was the recurring observation that within 10 to 20 minutes, each child used a few toys to express some disturbing fact of his life or some life task. In his studies of the same children over time, performances were characterized by a continuity of themes. Erikson remarked that "it is a common experience, and yet always astounding that all but the most inhibited children go at such a task with a peculiar eagerness" (p. 128). And further, that "there follows an absorption in the selection of toys, in the placement of blocks, and in the grouping of dolls which soon seems to follow some imperative theme" (128). After analyzing children's play from both cross-sectional and longitudinal vantage points, Erikson concluded:

> The themes presented betray some repetitiousness which we recognize as the "working through" of a *traumatic* experience: but they also express a playful *renewal*. If they seem to be governed by some need to *communicate*, or even to *confess*, they certainly also serve the joy of *self-expression*. If they seem dedicated to the *exercise* of growing facilities, they also seem to serve the *mastery* of a complex life situation. (p. 131)

The mastery-building experiences affirmed by creative, goal-directed, and fantasy play activity are almost as essential to the organism as sustenance through food. This was highlighted by Anna Freud (1965) in her conclusion:

Proficiency and pleasure in games are, thus, a complex achievement, dependent on contributions from many areas of the child's personality such as the endowment and intactness of the motor apparatus; a positive cathexis to the body and its skills; acceptance of companionship and group life; positive employment of controlled aggression in the service of ambition, etc. (p. 83)

With the handicapped child, or the child who has experienced severe emotional deprivation, one often notes an inability to master the developmental achievements which clearly depend on critical periods (Piaget, 1972; Van der Kooiz, 1977). Deficiencies in play lead to dysfunctional leisure and recreation behavior, while the development of play skills leads to mastery over the experiences of failure and the strengthening of a sense of hope (Erikson, 1963). The effect is an insidious lack of the *kinds* of experiences which children need, and which lead to expectations that reaching out, manipulating, experimenting and exploring with people and things can bring pleasant results. The importance of play as a precursor of later development was noted by Bettleheim (1965):

No child can enjoy an adequate social life unless he has acquired the ability to play with other children. Play, much more than adult-imposed learning, is the area where the child tests and develops his independence, where he learns to hold his own with his peers. (p. 198)

GUIDELINES FOR PLANNING A THERAPEUTIC RECREATION PROGRAM

The 1981 Joint Commission on Accreditation of Hospitals' *Consolidated Standards Manual* was designed to assess the quality of health care services in the United States.

The section of this document which relates to recreation and leisure services for children and adolescents includes the following:

1. A plan shall be written which describes the organization of the activity service or arrangements;
2. The goals and objectives of the services shall be stated in writing;

3. Appropriate activities shall be provided during the day, in the evening and on weekends;
4. Activity services shall be incorporated into the treatment plans — they shall reflect an assessment of individual needs, interest, life experiences, capacities and deficiencies;
5. Individual records shall contain progress notes that describe response to activity services and other pertinent observations; and
6. Appropriate space, equipment and facilities shall be provided to meet the activity service needs of individuals.

In a similar vein, the 1974 JCAH *Accreditation Manual for Psychiatric Facilities Servicing Children and Adolescents* specified that recreational and social activities:

1. shall be planned to aid the nature of each child's individuality, creativity, learning, motor, cognitive, and social skills — integrating these into a positive sense of self;
2. shall be planned so that children have opportunities to interact with others of different ages and of both sexes and to develop new interests and skills that help them gain self-confidence and acceptance by others;
3. shall be a balance of active group play, competitive endeavors, and quiet, solitary activities made for the provision of such services;
4. should provide opportunities to participate in normal community activities as they are able, including, where necessary, the transportation and supervision required for maximum usage of general community resources as appropriate, and
5. that initiation and termination of participation in any activity shall be timed in accordance with individual needs and ability to tolerate one activity for a period of time.

A minimum requirement for recreation and leisure programming for handicapped youth is adherence to the standard goal-setting procedures mandated by P.L. 94-142. The following steps, when implemented, offer marked advantages over services which look upon play as being of secondary significance and not part of habilitative efforts. As a legitimate therapeutic and educational tool, recreation and leisure activities should include the following:

1. *Establishment of each child's baseline level of skill.* Staff members observe the child's play in a variety of settings and times to arrive at statements of typical performance. A standard set of developmental scales describing characteristics of recreation and leisure skills is crucial. Wehman and Schleien (1981) identified 21 such scales to assess leisure skill competencies and potentials which are useful for handicapped populations. These measures are directed toward identification of features such as: proficiency with which objects or materials are engaged, length of self-initiated action, materials preference by clients, and frequency and direction of social interactions.

2. *Matching activities to needs.* Staff members decide on the growth priorities of each child. Based on observed readiness levels (earlier developmental tasks deemed mastered), activities are introduced which are appropriate to the child's capabilities and limitations.

3. *Specification of goals and objectives.* Staff members establish criteria for mastery of objectives. Ideally, ratings should focus on whether the child accomplishes the criteria under specified task conditions, for example, John will work on a 50 piece jigsaw puzzle for at least 50 minutes, with at least 5 correct fits, 80% of the time. Mager (1976) suggested that such behaviorally stated instructional objectives should involve three basic components: (a) a statement of given conditions under which the targeted performance should occur, (b) a description of the desired performance, and (c) a statement of the criterion for adequate performance.

4. *Measuring growth.* Growth may be charted as the number or percentage of objectives mastered within a specific period of time. Analysis of behavior change, or lack of change, provides feedback to assess each child's successes or failures in specific areas. The staff makes necessary program adjustments such as setting new objectives or modifying the complexity of the activity. Following this analysis, the cycle begins again with step 1 above.

The development of curriculae to build leisure and recreational skills in handicapped children is an outgrowth of early efforts to build self-help and language skills. Deinstitutionalization, Least Restrictive Environment, and normalization goals have led to greater efforts to identify effective approaches in these areas. Two distinctly different leisure skill training methods for disabled individuals have emerged: the developmental approach and the functional approach.

The developmental approach is characterized by identifying tasks along a continuum of age equivalents. For example, tasks vary from simple motor skills at the preschool level (i.e., grasping an object), to more advanced adolescent-level social skills (i.e., making telephone calls). Wehman and Schleien (1981), strong proponents of the principle of normalization as a guiding force in programming for handicapped individuals, noted that most handicapped individuals are developmentally immature in one or more curriculum areas. They advocate the use of child development norms in selecting and sequencing instructional content of skill building curriculae "to gradually reduce the differentness in performance of disabled persons while simultaneously expanding the public's degree of acceptance of their differentness" (p. 6).

The functional approach is characterized by identifying specific instructional objectives which lead to the generation of skill sequences in a step-by-step fashion. By deriving the component skills of the objectives, and eliminating unnecessary and redundant components, a hierarchy is established for each training objective. For example, making a peanut butter and jelly sandwich, after a task analysis, may be broken down into 12 separate steps, beginning with "grasp jar of peanut butter with nondominant hand, using palmar grasp" and concluding with "line up both slices of bread to complete sandwich" (p. 103).

A review of existing literature about leisure and recreational training programs suggests that both types of approaches are useful in providing educators and parents with guidelines necessary for coherent curriculum building and implementation.

With this brief theoretical background, the balance of the paper will deal with general approaches for developing effective recreation and leisure services for handicapped children.

GENERAL ACTIVITY PROGRAMMING GOALS FOR HANDICAPPED YOUTH

Successful activity programming, even where such activity is largely spontaneous, often rests on careful planning by adults.

Whether the games and pastimes of youth provide a sense of pleasure to their participants depends in large measure on factors of appropriate grouping, materials, space, knowledge, and mental images of play activity. Habilitation for handicapped youngsters, through activity programming, must anticipate and control peer rejection, lack of interpersonal awareness, and lack of self-control (Gottman et al., 1975; Ross & Bernstein, 1976; Rinn & Markle, 1979; Goodman & Miller, 1980; Eisler & Fredericksen, 1980).

Few of the frequently quoted purposes for including recreation in school and treatment settings will be realized unless the activities are *designed* to accommodate to and promote certain social and emotional behaviors. Whether we speak of music appreciation, a museum trip, jogging, video games, an arts and crafts project, simple board or card games, or competitive sports, an analysis of "game" features is essential (Lament, 1978; Marlowe, 1980). Game features include specifications of required equipment, movements, organizational patterns, purpose, and participants. The guiding adult must become aware of, and be prepared to assume responsibility for, the different aspects of each game or activity (Quilitch, 1977; Rumanoff, 1978).

The following social and emotional experiences, though incomplete, may be viewed as general guidelines for setting goals for the planned activity of handicapped children. They deal with conditions that are necessary for enlarging children's capacity to learn and to sustain their growth-producing experiences.

Involvement

The handicapped child frequently has not developed sufficient skill (attention, confidence, etc.) to approach and master his environment. Hewett and Forness (1984) emphasized the necessity of getting a child to attend to, and participate in, activities as a prerequisite for mastery of higher order competencies. Engagement in a purposeful activity is fundamental to any learning and to any corrective emotional experience. When stimuli appear to be too confusing or threatening, physical and/or emotional withdrawal usually occurs. Security needs take precedence over exploratory needs. Such children tend to experience situations in a passive rather than active manner. Stereotyped avoidance or feelings of boredom characterize the behavioral styles of many handicapped children.

To help these children overcome their reluctance to become involved, adults must prepare environments that are perceived as safe. Techniques successfully used to reduce excessive emotional responses include desensitization, simplification of task demands, prompting (i.e., physical guidance to establish response), fading (i.e., gradual removal of physical guidance), and introduction of behavior models (Bandura & Walters, 1963; Flavell, 1973; Perry & Cerreto, 1977; Wehman, 1977; Wehman & Schleien, 1981).

A system of appropriate positive reinforcements helps to sustain involvement once it has begun. Paloutzian et al., (1971) demonstrated that severely retarded young institutionalized children could learn to imitate, and that simple imitative repertoires could be extended to include relatively complex social repertoires. A significantly higher level of social behavior was demonstrated by children who received imitative training than children who were not trained to imitate, based on staff scoring of a social interaction rating scale. Imitative training consisted of sitting opposite the child and requesting "do this" with arm, face, hand or foot gestures. Prompting (physical guidance of the child's body) was added if the child did not respond within a specified time period. When (either non-aided or aided) imitative responses were produced, the child received both verbal praise ("good boy") and a food reinforcer (a spoonful of ice cream). After gradual fading of physical prompts, the trained group subsequently demonstrated increased social responsiveness.

Strain (1975) demonstrated that social repertoires of withdrawn, severely retarded preschool children could be significantly increased through operant training procedures. Teachers read familiar stories (The Three Bears, Red Riding Hood, Snow White, etc.) during 15 minute story-time periods in a developmental nursery school, and assigned socio-dramatic roles to the children. Teachers modeled and prompted them to imitate appropriate role behaviors of their assigned character, offering contingent verbal praise on a continuous reinforcement schedule. The children produced significant increases in social play during rest of the day play periods, for instance, sharing roles, as in playing store, fireman, etc., building on the same structure, taking turns on play equipment, holding hands, handing objects to peers, etc. When compared with eight days of baseline observations which were characterized by low, stable amounts of social play, twelve days of socio-dramatic training produced rapid acceleration of social play. When socio-dramatic play training was terminated, there was an immediate deceleration of social play. An immediate increase in the level of social play after resumption of socio-dramatic training (reversal design) demonstrated that basic operant training techniques are easily adapted into preschool routines and require less teacher time and less active monitoring of child behavior than intervention strategies utilizing contingent edible reinforcement. This is particularly important when dealing simultaneously with target behavior of several handicapped children.

Competition and Cooperation

Competitiveness normally arises from an internalization of cultural values, and from a desire to excel. At about age three or four, children start to exhibit rivalry over possessions and over the affection and attention of adults. We know that almost all handicapped children, regardless of type or level of disability, have significant deficits in capacity for competitive and cooperative interaction. The deficits experienced in cognitive, language and self-help areas lead to a failure syndrome. If uncorrected, they may result in subsequent adjustment problems ranging from apathy and avoidance to delinquency (Roff et al., 1972; Kelly 1982). Children with such handicaps withdraw from competitive social interaction. This sets the stage for self-defeating patterns of social and emotional skill deficits. Recreational activity, when monitored and controlled, can provide safe and pleasurable forms of competition and promote a more positive self-concept (Ausubel, 1958; Wambold & Bailey, 1979).

Cooperation requires a higher level of maturity than competition. It presumes a capacity for subordinating one's own primitive needs and an ability to differentiate role behavior. Age-appropriate projects such as planting and maintaining flower gardens, making props for a play and decorating bulletin boards are examples of planned, joint activities between handicapped and nonhandicapped peers. Sailor and Haring (1977), Wehman and Marchant (1978), Wehman

(1979), and Brown et al. (1979), have reported training programs to decrease such behaviors as refusal to play, lack of sustained play, throwing toys, etc., and to build appropriate cooperative, sharing behaviors. Studies of programs which provide opportunities for play between severely handicapped and nonhandicapped children indicate trends toward successful integration. They indicate that competitive and cooperative skills can be developed even in severely handicapped youngsters (Salend, 1981). Recreational activities designed to move children from isolate play into differentiated social roles play a paramount role in any curriculum for socialization.

Morris and Dolker (1974) noted that the teaching of cooperative skills is of major importance in any therapeutic program for retarded children, and that the absence of such skills distinguishes the severely retarded from higher level retardates. They concluded from their experimental studies of play enhancement that patterns of withdrawal and low social interaction in retarded children may be due not only to a paucity of reinforcement for social interaction and cooperative play, but also to the absence of socially interactive and reinforcing role models. In a study of six nonverbal, withdrawn retarded children ages four through twelve, all with measurable IQs below 30, the experimenters demonstrated that cooperative play (i.e., rolling a ball between two children seated on the floor, facing each other) could be significantly increased when the withdrawn children were paired with "highly interactive" retarded child "helpers." Their findings indicated that high-low interactive child pairs improved significantly from baseline play levels after 1-1/2 hours of training. Such training included physical guidance, praise, and candy reinforcers for completion of reciprocal ball-rolling. Results showed that having high interactive child models was a major factor in improvement of low interactive children, and yielded higher gains than when two low interactive children were trained as pairs, or when a low interactive child was trained under isolate shaping conditions with an adult evaluator.

Marchant and Wehman (1979) concluded that severely retarded children can acquire simple cooperative table game skills in a relatively brief period of time provided the skills are taught in a systematic manner. Four children, ages eight to ten, with mental age equivalents of 21 to 46 months (three of whom were nonverbal), acquired 80% of the steps designed to teach them mastery of a lotto game. The game was adapted to make handling of the cards a less difficult motor task. An example of the steps involved in one of the cooperative games is the following nine step task analysis of a three card lotto game: (a) child stacks cards in pile, (b) player 1 draws a card from stack and matches to corresponding illustration. If card is not a match, it will be placed in a new stack, (c) player 2 does step 2, (d) play continues until one person has all three cards matched and wins, (e) number of starting cards increased to six, (f) child plays with adult, (g) child plays with both a child and an adult, (h) child plays with child under adult supervision, (i) child plays with another child independently. Parents of children participating in the training indicated that skills were transferred and maintained as reflected by the fact that the children showed increased rates of independent game play at home. Sequences like the one just listed may be preceded by prerequisite training steps if necessary, such as: (a) extend dominant hand toward stack of cards; (b) grasp top card using pincer grasp; (c) rotate wrist until face of card is in view; (d) identify picture on card; (e) match picture to appropriate picture on game board; (f) release first card into space by extending fingers; (g) match second card to appropriate board space; (h) match third and subsequent cards to game board spaces until all spaces are covered (Wehman & Schleien, 1981).

Independence

One of the long-term goals of basic education is the emergence of an independent individual. Development of the self as a stable and independent entity occurs when activities reinforce a notion of mastery. Peer values are learned through internalization of the rules and rituals of recreational play. It provides a source of derived status and helps to reduce dependency upon adults. Security-giving adults, in their turn, are replaced as essential socializing agents as mastery experiences accumulate. Mastery over recreational activities typically progresses from early stages in which the child is largely dependent on reinforcement from others, to involvement in recreation and leisure experiences. This typically leads to acquisition of status through independent accomplishment (Marion, 1979; Sabatino & Schloss, 1981).

Developing a child's self-reliance is at the opposite pole from promoting his involvement in the environment. Challenging physical activities, such as traversing a rope course, are inherently reinforcing. They can be used to help handicapped youngsters gain a fuller understanding of their own resources and strengths. Adventure recreation departs from individual or team competition. Activities requiring the effort of all group members not only help to develop a sense of group membership, they stimulate positive feelings of accomplishment and esteem.

Children need opportunities to practice a variety of roles in order to exercise independence, self direction, and decision making. Ego development in this area can be fostered through the availability of such experiences as offered in recreation and leisure activity.

UNDERSTANDING AND MEETING THE RECREATION AND LEISURE NEEDS OF HANDICAPPED YOUTH

The social-emotional needs and characteristics of handicapped youth differ in degree but not in kind from the general population. That is, the major and minor behavioral disabilities found among the general population are also found to occur in handicapped populations. However, social-emotional deficits occur more *frequently* among the handicapped group (Gardner, 1977). Specific causal relationships between handicapping conditions (skill deficits) and behavior disturbances cannot be assumed. However, programs directed at improving the social competence of handicapped children, and offering them greater involvement in areas of normal functioning, may reduce conditions which support dysfunctional behavior. This concept is at the heart of the Least Restrictive Environment philosophy (Rehmann & Riggen, 1977; Dybwad, 1982). According to the Education of All Handicapped Children Act of 1975 (P.L.94-142), separation of handicapped children into special service programs is permissable only when the handicaps are of such a nature that the child could *not* be taught or managed satisfactorily in regular programs. This provision makes good educational sense, but its full implementation presents unique challenges to those responsible for adapting existing resources to meet the needs of handicapped children.

The sense of inadequacy, inferiority, and vulnerability often seen in these children sets the stage for adult overprotection and peer rejection (Mercer, 1971; Schloss, 1982). Reduced social opportunities perpetuate low self-esteem and low peer acceptance. Recreation and leisure resources for handicapped youth need to be utilized to counteract previous negative social experiences.

The special needs of these children require the establishment of specific objectives. Educational and therapeutic programs endorse the notion that successes experienced in recreation and leisure activities will meet the child's needs for (a) emotional development and his sense of self, (b) social development and his sense of relatedness, (c) motoric development and his sense of vitality, (d) cognitive development and his thinking/knowledge base, and (e) communication development and his receptive/expressive language skills. Each of these needs is briefly discussed below.

Emotional Development and the Sense of Self

Each child develops his unique style for dealing with tension, frustration, fear, and other unpleasant feelings. The handicapped child, often with poorer internal controls, and with fewer successful adaptive behavior patterns, is subject to more emotional problems than other normal children his age (Michelson & Wood, 1980; Kelly, 1982). His self-esteem is poorer. His confidence is lower. Recreational activities can give a youngster the feeling of success, a product to show off, a performance to be proud of, and a sense of belonging to a group. For example, adventure activities can develop a stronger sense of self and provide a basis to overcome chronic feelings of vulnerability and compensate for a sense of helplessness (Frant et al., 1985).

Social Development and the Sense of Relatedness

The social withdrawal patterns of handicapped children, and experiences of rejection by their more competent peers and/or adults, are widely recognized phenomena (Bryan, 1974). Research studies reporting on the interactions of handicapped and nonhandicapped children in integrated settings have found fewer positive social interactions for the former group. Nondisabled children more frequently initiated eye gaze toward, smiled at, touched, vocalized to, sat next to, and chose as playmates *other* nondisabled children than they did disabled classmates (Guralnick, 1980; Peterson, 1982). Since the passage of P.L.94-142, handicapped youngsters have been integrated into more mainstream activities. This heightens the need for development of their social skills. If social skill deficits are not modified, handicapped children will not experience sufficient success to develop more advanced social skills. Withdrawal and other inappropriate behaviors will become increasingly debilitating and deepen the sense of isolation from peers.

The basic social skills needed for relating to peers can best be observed and reinforced during recreational activity. Some of these skills are (a) ability to demonstrate behaviors which reinforce peers (giving compliments, offering to share, following rules, etc.); (b) responding appropriately to peer initiated behavior; and (c) staying in close physical proximity to peers. Techniques for improving these social skills have appeared in the growing literature of social learning theory and behavior modification (Gardner, 1977; Strain, 1982; Schloss, 1982; Hewett & Forness, 1984). Eisler and Fredericksen (1980) described a social skill training program which could be used with handicapped children to build a repertoire of prosocial skills during play. An example follows:

> Scott needs basic training in initiating social activities, and in learning how to engage in cooperative play. For purposes of effective training, we must break these general skills into more specific components. Thus, for Scott to initiate social activities, he must first learn how to look and smile at other children in a friendly manner. He must also learn how, verbally and nonverbally, to indicate to the other children that he desires to engage in a particular social activity.
>
> Trainer: One of the best ways I know to make friends is to smile at people like this (*trainer smiles*). Do you think you could smile when you look at me?
> Scott: Like this? (*smiles*)
> Trainer: Yes, that's very good Scott. Let's see you do it again (*trainer smiles*).

After smiling has been practiced with the trainer for awhile, Scott is asked to practice smiling first at his teacher and then at another child. Once Scott has mastered this with a number of other children, training is begun on the next skill, offering to share toys.

Trainer: One of the best ways to make friends is to share one of your favorite toys with them in a game. Do you have any toys that you think the other children would like to play with? Scott: I have a big red fire truck.
Trainer: Let's call Andy over here to see if he wants to play with your fire truck. Watch how to do this Scott. "Hey Andy, want to come over here and play with my truck?"
Andy: How does it work?
Trainer: Scott, why don't you show Andy how it works?

. . . The trainer must initially be very much involved in structuring the practice with others and then gradually withdraw his involvement when it becomes apparent that the child can perform under these circumstances, and the natural responses of others will maintain the new behavior.

. . . Individualized training approaches utilizing coaching, modeling, and feedback can be employed during the role-playing of socially skilled responses. (pp. 170-171)

Since the passage of P.L. 94-142, handicapped youngsters have been involved in more mainstream activities. This heightens the need for early development of their social skills. Such skills can be trained and reinforced in the child's natural environment.

Motoric Development and the Sense of Vitality

Anyone who has watched children in active play has seen that those who exhibit higher levels of motor skills are more popular with their peer group than those who have few skills. The playground is a major arena for demonstration of motor coordination, balance, strength, agility, and speed. Although children with mild levels of handicap often have the least difficulty of being integrated with their normal peers, even those with severe physical disability can experience success in active group participation (Sirvis & Cieloha, 1981). Decisions can be made about possible needs for adaptive equipment after reviewing the capabilities of the child involved with regard to his interests and his capacity for controlled movements, strength, mobility, and balance. Some examples of adaptive materials for handicapped children include (a) short badminton racket handles which offer easier handling, (b) handles wrapped with a sponge and tape for easier gripping, (c) adjusted height and diameter of basketball hoops to suit the ability level of participants, (d) beanbags instead of soft balls to make catching easier, (e) balloons instead of balls when first learning to catch because of their slow flight, (f) adjustable batting tee or ball suspended from the ceiling to teach hitting, (g) sledding disks preliminary to sleds with runners, and (h) handle grip bowling balls, etc.

A child's ability to be vitally and confidently involved in play is a most important component in normalization. Conversely, motor incompetence acts as a limiting factor in competitive and cooperative peer activities (Humberman, 1976; Sherrill, 1976). Mastery of swimming, biking, running, skating, etc., can provide feelings of exhilaration in both solitary and group activities.

Cognitive Development and Thinking/Knowledge Base

No significant or lasting effect on cognitive development has been found after encouraging children to engage in activities such as drawing, jumping, bouncing, crawling etc. (Hammill et al. (1974). Meyen (1982) concluded that while perceptual motor skills are necessary for acceptance in the child's peer group, they cannot be a substitute for cognitive development through academic instruction. Still, play and recreation activity may help handicapped children to learn more efficiently when they produce increased task motivation and attention. Games which are specifically selected to encourage children to notice, examine, see relationships, evaluate, and make decisions (card and board games, circle games, etc.) stimulate thinking about the environment. Games as learning tools have long been used to promote concept formation. The evolution of the computer and availability of simulation games, provide significant additions to the storehouse of recreation and leisure possibilities (Rushakoff & Lombardino, 1983).

Communication Development and Receptive/Expressive Language Skills

Nonverbal and social skill prerequisites of purposeful and effective communication are frequently delayed or deficient in handicapped children. The normal model of language development is widely accepted in practice as the basis for improving communication skills. Typically, the first order of business focuses on social skills. The following can be learned through modeling and reinforcement in play and recreation settings: eye contact, mutual eye gaze, active listening to a partner, nonverbal gestures of intent, facial expressions to relate feelings, and body position with appropriate social distance. Once these are present, recreational activities can facilitate higher order communication skills such as verbal turntaking, giving sufficient information, using specific vocabulary for description, and the ability to ask relevant questions, etc., (Whitehill et al., 1980; Bates, 1980).

Teaching through group play is an excellent vehicle for developing the above skills. Heterogeneous group composition ideally presents the communication handicapped child with playmates who have more advanced communication skills. Recreational activities to promote modeling of good communication skills include dollhouse play, mural painting, pantomime, creative dramatics, puppetry, etc. (Strain, 1982)

Successful experiences in the six areas noted above should provide the handicapped child with a sense of unity which can set the stage for greater actualization of his potential.

PRACTICAL APPLICATIONS OF THERAPEUTIC RECREATION AND LEISURE PROGRAMS

In this paper, activities included under *play* cover the range from solitary *playfulness* (repetitive patterns of pleasureful behavior) to *organized recreation* (goal-directed group interaction). Preceding sections alluded to the habilitative effects of recreation and leisure on the ego. Capacity for feedback and self-correction are the attributes of the ego which make leisure and recreational programming a vital therapeutic tool. By offering opportunities for play and by reinforcing appropriate play with social recognition and approval, a child's capacity for joy and self-actualization is increased. For handicapped youngsters, barriers to success may dissolve through fantasy activity, and boundaries which previously excluded him can dissolve.

Mundy and Odum (1979) have advocated a continuum of developmental skills beginning with leisure awareness, progressing through social and recreation skills, and terminating in exploration and usage of community resources for recreational fulfillment.

The models presented next are arranged in order of applicability to children and adolescents with three different levels of handicap; profound, moderate to severe, and mild. They have in common a developmental design to help handicapped youth experience their humanity through play, recreation and leisure.

Profoundly Handicapped Students

Central to the social-emotional and cognitive disturbances of profoundly handicapped children is a communication and motivational defect so severe that their capacity to form relationships is critically impaired. Kaufman's (1975, 1981) patient and intense involvement with his own autistic son is a touching example of work with a profoundly handicapped child. He transmitted his sense of profound joy when observing the child's sense of discovery, excitement, and pleasure in play, especially when that same child was previously mired in impotent activity, confusion, and hopelessness. For this type of child, differentiation of the affective quality of interaction is typically absent or profoundly limited. It is as if the child finds no rewards in being with and relating to people. Interaction is confused and erratic because his definition of self in relation to others is unclear. The child does not know how to use the human environment. This often indicates a breakdown in ego functioning during the period in early childhood when play is supposed to establish a sense of interpersonal roles, and the way people feel and behave.

The literature on successful efforts to change broad patterns of profound emotional disturbance is not encouraging. At primitive levels of ego-functioning, treatment models have generally stressed intense one-to-one interaction. Group-oriented approaches have limited applicability at this level. Recreation and leisure programming must be postponed until more basic skills in the hierarchy of interaction and self-awareness are established.

A primary goal with this population is the development of improved human awareness and relationships through encouragement of close and intimate physical contact. One such program developed by DesLauriers (1965) is described under the general name "theraplay." In theraplay, there are no toys, objects or games. The instruments of contact with the child are the adults themselves, with their intrusive, constant and persistent presence. The worker asserts him/herself in an actively playful and exciting way, and becomes the central instrument of contact and communication of feeling. Through the direct physical and sensory stimulation of theraplay, the child is led to (a) find pleasure in human contact, (b) discover his own body and its functions, (c) seek increased and more varied human contacts in the pursuit of his basic needs, (d) derive joy in his own activities and accomplishments, (e) sense connectedness with others, and (f) initiate simple problem-solving behaviors. In theraplay, then, the child is encouraged to progressively grow toward a world that is not frightening even though it is demanding and challenging.

Any teacher, child care worker, or therapist seriously interested in working with profoundly disturbed children should be thoroughly conversant with levels of play interaction described by DesLauriers:

1. "Being With": The adult attempts to be in the presence of the child under conditions which cause him no discomfort. The child should not be disorganized by unnecessary movements, and should be kept at a distance that is neither too close nor too far away.
2. "Moving With": The adult imitates or follows the child's movements, so that both parties experience a heightened awareness of each other.
3. "Playing With": The adult *parallels* the movements of the child in order to stimulate social activity where a child's social repertoire is quite limited.
4. "Signing With": By bodily communication and activity, the adult moves toward attempting to communicate intention or need.

5. "Music With": The adult incorporates rhythm to involve the child in joint goal-directed activity.
6. "Speech With": Using reinforcers, adults attempt to introduce speech to promote communication and play activity.

At the level of profound handicap, techniques of ego reconstruction through play are designed to promote visual and physical contact (Hingtgen & Bryson, 1972). Parallel physical activity, or synchronism, is designed to lead to a heightened awareness of self and significant others.

Moderately-Severely Handicapped Students

Space, time, and behavior structures must be built into any interpersonal system if it is to result in an effective social environment for youth with moderate-to-severe social, emotional, or cognitive handicaps (Turner, Hersen, & Bellack, 1978). Limitation of space deals with *where* a child responds, and reduces potential for distraction and off-target wandering. The time structure focuses on the attention-span demands and specification of *when* a child is to respond. The behavior structure identifies the *what* (rather than the *how well*) of acceptable responses.

Many children at this level act as if their inner lives (thoughts, feelings, perceptions, etc.) are chaotic and disorganized. Play activity, arranged in an orderly, sequentially sound, and well-organized manner, provides a compensatory external simplification of the environment. The behavior of children functioning at a primitive social level must be under the immediate control of the change agent. To develop a sense of internal order in handicapped children, adults must introduce external order. Redl (1972) noted:

> We have plenty of evidence now that, other things being equal, the very exposure of children to a given game, with its structure and demands for certain constituent performances, may have terrific clinical effect. . . . Whenever we miscalculate the overwhelming effects that the seductive aspect of certain games may have, we may ask for trouble, whereas many a seemingly risky game can be safely played if enough ego-supportive controls are built into it. (p. 87)

If recreational and leisure demands are geared to a level of auditory, visual, perceptual, memory, language, cognitive, and/or motor skills which are beyond the child's capability at the time, program objectives will not be met. The interest and activity levels of non-disabled peers should serve as models of the desired recreational behavior. Such an approach offers opportunities for the handicapped child to improve his skills, and for the normal peer to appreciate the learning by his playmate (Wehman & Schleien, 1981). Selection of activities should, of course, be appealing to the children and geared to their interest.

Two useful criterion-referenced models which provide hierarchies of play skills integrated with prescriptive teaching programs are the *Experimental Curriculum for Young Retarded Children* by Connor and Talbot (1970), and the *Behavioral Characteristics Progression Program* by Wickersham and Bland (1977).

The Connor and Talbot program provides a step by step curriculum guide with specific instructions to teachers to initiate goal-directed action by handicapped children and to immediately reinforce them. This prescriptive model is based on (a) the breakdown of content into small steps, (b) the prompting of successive steps toward mastery of objectives, and (c) the gradual disappearance of prompts as the autonomy of the child becomes evident. The skill training programs were designed to be applied during "discussion periods, handwork activities, story telling, music experiences, juice time, free play sessions, motor activities, swimming, cooking, and trips" (p. 6).

Wickersham and Bland provide an effective planning and evaluation tool in their BCP program which features a comprehensive listing of behavioral objectives for individualized teaching. Behavioral objectives on the BCP are designed to match pupil educational needs in five domains: Self-Help (nine skills), Motor (twelve skills), Communication (eleven skills), Social (six skills), and Learning (six skills). Both models set up a continuum of behavior competencies in specific adaptive functions. One can use these models to develop prerequisite skills necessary for successful play by (a) identifying the child's *current* level of skill along a specific strand or dimension, (b) identifying the *next* skills in the developmental sequences selected for the child to master, and (c) specifying task conditions and behavior levels for demonstration of mastery at the target level. For example, in the Music and Rhythm area of the BCP, there are 34 developmental steps. The sequence begins with "mimics simple, gross hand movements (e.g., claps with music)," continues through ten steps to "participates in group songs with singing voice," and through ten more steps to "plays rhythm instrument in simple pattern." Both the Connor-Talbot and the Wickersham-Bland models give precise teaching strategies to help youth attain targeted skill levels. In this way, skill objectives are selected, staff functions clarified and child progress measured. Examples of some BCP recreation skills applicable to a handicapped population include such diverse areas as Arts and Crafts, Outdoor Skills, Swimming, etc. Related adaptive skill areas which should be incorporated in an overall program include Impulse Control, Visual-Motor Skills, Gross Motor Skills, Social Eating, Social Speech, Interpersonal Relations, etc.

Mildly Handicapped Students

The largest percentage of handicapped children and adolescents falls into this group. This is a population which, at maturity, should be able to attain a more or less independent lifestyle. The ultimate attainment of independence seems more likely to impact on social-emotional maturity than upon cognitive skill achievements. Overcoming a poor self-concept, low frustration tolerance, and a sense of social alienation are some of the objectives addressed in therapeutic recreation programming.

Most youngsters with handicaps at this level have the capacity to master fairly complex interpersonal recreation skills. Structured learning programs which use behavioral techniques of contracting, modeling, and social reinforcement have proven successful in several areas of social skill development (i.e., participation, assertiveness, etc. (Schloss, 1984).

To promote the acquisition of critical life skills *including* recreation and leisure skills, the author has developed several programs for mildly handicapped (mildly mentally retarded, learning disabled, perceptually impaired, and socially maladjusted) adolescents. These programs identify behavior skills in four domains:

Academic-Vocational, Personal, Self-help, and Social. Based on the Gunzburg *Process Assessment Chart* (for moderately retarded children and adults), and similar to the Connor-Talbot and the Wickersham-Bland models, these programs rely on specific skill challenges and reinforcement for success. The author's strategy for reducing adolescent resistance to change focuses on renewable skill contracts under the umbrella of a "Rainbow," the acronym for *Res*idential *A*chievement *IN*ventory, *B*ehavior *O*bservation *W*heel. A fundamental concept is that *both* staff and child agree to follow a set of routines which reduce the risk of regressive emotional over-reaction and regression in order to develop a climate of psychological safety and security. Without such a climate, significant psychological growth toward self-confidence and interpersonal maturity is unlikely. The primary role of staff is to use the array of skills presented in the Rainbow chart to provide concrete objectives, where expectancies are operationally clear, and parallel the developmental dynamics of adolescent striving toward independence. Presented in this format, even handicapped adolescents may see more clearly that coming into adulthood is not an *event* heralded by a certain birthday or physical maturity, but rather, is the culmination of a *process* of mastering a series of status-giving social, emotional and cognitive skills.

The Rainbow program, comprised of more than 150 developmental tasks, can be used to promote confidence and hope when structured as short-term challenges. Recreational activities specified in the program involve youths in experiences with normal peers. Staff and the child independently rate that child's skill levels. After the ratings, they mutually designate the next month's objectives, i.e., the establishment of mastery in transitional and undeveloped skill areas. Ensuing discussion should assure that staff and student are mutually responsible for promoting success. Staff roles include the provision of proper materials, constructive advice and "hurdle help" when needed. As an example of one month's objectives, derived from three of the 24 Rainbow scales and, based on mastery of preceding skills, a student may be challenged to demonstrate the following behavior patterns:

Scale J Level 2 — Leisure Time Skills: Learns and/or regularly demonstrates the ability to participate in and have fun in at least three different games that can be played by 2 to 4 individuals, e.g., cards, dominoes, checkers, Monopoly, etc. Participates and shows capacity to complete 90% of games started with a spirit of fun.

Scale Q Level 2 — Competitive Skills: Regularly participates in situations which involve some competitive strain, and maintains ability to control primitive emotional outbursts, e.g., threatening, screaming, etc. When upset, able to terminate threatening behavior easily and without defiance after only one staff reminder at least 9 out of 10 times.

Scale R Level 3 — Cooperative Skills: Student takes initiative or accepts responsibility to help another student at least twice per week on a fairly intensive basis, e.g., homework, assigned undone chores, etc.

Successfully completed contracts are followed by appropriate extrinsic rewards, i.e., increased privileges, as well as social reinforcement, i.e., praise. As adolescents succeed at developmentally higher levels of tasks, they begin to feel more mature and able to *let go* of primitive, regressive, and delinquent modes of behavior. Goals and gains are recorded on a chart depicting the target skills of the program, and an updated copy is given to the student. Overly lenient credit on the Rainbow Chart is a poor substitute for the actual underlying skill, and inappropriate credit may actually impede progress and a desire for mastery. Mildly handicapped adolescents benefit from treatment systems that are developmentally relevant, provide challenging activities, and a sense of power over achievable objectives. This is in accordance with Josselyn's (1948) observation that "only by experiencing the satisfactions of independent and interdependent activities can youth resist the lure of permanent childhood" (p. 27).

Quite apart from the pleasureful and growth-inducing aspects of successful play, recreation and leisure activities also can assist in the experience of a sense of unity. The ability to act autonomously and to fill what Bettleheim calls the "in-between times" with goal-directed, prosocial activity is a distinguishing characteristic of growing maturity. Images of past successes, and feelings of mastery over feelings of boredom are powerful socializing effects. Creating an environment to facilitate such effects and to produce the social and emotional experiences which precede them, constitutes an undertaking of the first order in the educational treatment of handicapped children.

The importance of personal autonomy achieved through mastery in leisure skill areas is aptly described by Bettleheim (1965):

> The help the child needs in overcoming his fear in the next activity is not limited to bridging the in-between moments. A life that is divided into separate parts cannot easily make sense, hence it cannot be mastered. The in-between times must stop being empty spaces that separate disconnected actions. They must become sensible links in a sequence of events. They must convince the child of the unity of his life through the only example that is pervasive enough to force him to establish, in its image, the unity of his own personality. (p. 119)

Indeed, for many children, the sense of mastery in play and its derivatives may just be those images which best stimulate the child to experience himself as a unity. Through successful goal-directed play, one can ignite a sense of confidence in the child's movements, and a feeling of hope for pleasurable outcomes. The modality of recreation and leisure programming has often been the key to the symbolic birth of social skills in handicapped youth.

REFERENCES

Ausubel, D. (1958). *Theory and problems of child development*. New York: Grune and Stratton.

Bandura, A., & Walters. (1963). *Social learning and personality development*. New York: Rinehart and Winston.

Bartel, N., & Guskin, S. (1980). A handicap as a social phenomenon. In W. Cruickshank (Ed.), *Psychology of exceptional children and youth*. (pp. 45-73). Englewood Cliffs, NJ: Prentice-Hall.

Bates, P. (1980). The effectiveness of interpersonal skills training on the social skills acquisition of moderately and mildly retarded adults. *Journal of Applied Behavior Analysis, 13,* 237-248.

Bettleheim, B. (1965). *Love is not enough.* New York: Collier Books.

Brown, L., Branston, M., Baumgart, D., Vinvent, L., Falvey, M., & Schroeder, J. (1979). Utilizing the characteristics of a variety of current and subsequent least restrictive environments as factors in the development of curricular content for severely handicapped students. *AAESPH Review, 4,* 407-424.

Bruininks, R. (1974). Physical and motor development of retarded persons. In N. Ellis (Ed.), *International Review of Research in Mental Retardation.* New York: Academic Press.

Bryan, T. (1974). An observational analysis of classroom behaviors of children with learning disabilities. *Journal of Learning Disabilities, 7,* 26-34.

Connor, F., & Talbot, M. (1970). *An experimental curriculum for young mentally retarded children.* New York: Teacher's College Press.

DesLauriers, A. (1965). *Theraplay.* Devon, PA: Devereux Foundation, unpublished.

Dewey, J. (1956). *The child and the curriculum: The school and society.* Chicago: Phoenix Books.

Dybwad, G. (1982). Avoiding misconceptions of mainstreaming: The least restrictive environment and normalization. In N. West (Ed.), *Educating exceptional children.* Guilford, CT: Dushkin Publishing Group.

Eisler, R., & Fredericksen, L. (1980). *Perfecting social skills: A guide to interpersonal behavior development.* New York: Plenum Press.

Erikson, E. (1963). *Childhood and society.* New York: Norton.

Erikson, E. (1972). Play and actuality. In W. Piers (Ed.), *Play and development.* New York: Norton.

Flavell, J. (1973). Reduction of stereotypes by reinforcement of toy play. *Mental Retardation, 11,* 21-23.

Freud, A. (1965). *Normality and pathology in childhood: Assessment of development.* New York: International Universities Press.

Gardner, W. (1977). *Learning and behavior characteristics of exceptional children and youth.* Boston: Allyn and Bacon.

Goodman, L., & Miller, H. (1980). Mainstreaming: How teachers can make it work. *Journal of Research and Development in Education, 13,* 45-57.

Gordon, I. (1962). *Human development from birth through adolescence.* New York: Harper and Bros.

Gottman, J., Gonso, J., & Rasmussen, B. (1976). Social interaction, social competence and friendship in children. *Child Development, 46,* 709-716.

Guralnick, M. (1978). *Early intervention and the integration of handicapped and nonhandicapped children.* Baltimore: University Park Press.

Guralnick, M. (1980). Social interactions among preschool children. *Exceptional children, 46,* 248-253.

Hammill, D., Goodman, L., & Wiederholt, J. (1974). Visual-motor processes: Can we trust them? *Reading Teacher, 27,* 469-486.

Hewett, F., & Forness, S. (1984). *Education of exceptional learners, 3rd edition.* Boston: Allyn and Bacon.

Hingtgen, J., & Bryson, C. (1972). Recent developments in the study of early childhood psychosis: Infantile autism, childhood schizophrenia and related disorders. *Schizophrenia bulletin, 5,* 8-53.

Humberman, G. (1976). Organized sports activities with cerebral palsied adolescents. *Rehabilitation Literature, 37*(4), 103-106.

Joint Commission on Accreditation of Hospitals. (1974). *Accreditation manual for psychiatric facilities serving children and adolescents.* Chicago.

Joint Commission on Accreditation of Hospitals. (1981). *Consolidated standards manual.* Chicago.

Josselyn, I. M. (1948). *Psychosocial development of children.* New York: Family Service Association of America.

Kaufman, B. (1976). *Son rise.* New York: Warner Books.

Kaufman, B. (1981). *A miracle to believe in.* New York: Fawcett Crest.

Kelly, J. (1982). *Social skills training: A practical guide to intervention.* New York: Springer.

Kooiz, R. van der, & Groot, R. de (1977). *That's all in the game: Theory and research, practice and future of childrens' play.* Rheinstetten: Schindele Verlag.

Lament, M. M. (1978). Reaching the exceptional student through music in the elementary classroom. *Teaching Exceptional Children, 11*(11), 32-38.

Marchant, J., & Wehman, P. (1979). Teaching table games to severely handicapped students. *Mental Retardation, 17,* 150-152.

Marion, R. L. (1979). Leisure time activities for trainable mentally retarded adolescents. *Teaching Exceptional Children, 11*(4), 158-161.

Marlowe, M. (1980). Games analysis: Designing games for handicapped children. *Teaching Exceptional Children, 12*(2), 48-50.

Mercer, J. (1971). The meaning of mental retardation. In R. Koch, & J. Dobson (Eds.), *The mentally retarded child and his family.* New York: Brunner/Mazel.

Meyen, E. (1982). *Exceptional children and youth.* Chicago: Love Publishing.

Michelson, L., & Wood, R. (1980). Behavioral assessment and training of children's social skills. In M. Herson, P. Miller, & R. Eisler (Eds.), *Progress in behavior modification.* New York: Academic Press.

Mager, R. (1976). *Preparing instructional objectives.* Belmont, CA: Fearon Publishers.

Morris, R., & Dolker, M. (1974). Developing cooperative play in socially withdrawn retarded children. *Mental Retardation, 12,* 24-27.

Mundy, J., & Odum, L. (1979). *Leisure education: Theory and practice.* New York: John Wiley.

Murphy, L. (1972). Infants' play and cognitive development. In W. Piers (Ed.), *Play and development.* New York: Norton.

Paloutzian, R. F., Hasazi, J., Streifel, J., & Edgar, C. (1971). Promotion of positive social interaction in severely retarded young children. *American Journal of Mental Deficiency, 75,* 519-524.

Perry, M., & Cerreto, M. (1977). Structured learning training of social skills for the retarded. *Mental Retardation, 15,* 31-33.

Peterson, N. (1982). Social interaction of handicapped and nonhandicapped preschoolers: A study of playmate preferences. *Topics in early childhood special education, 2,* 56-69.

Piaget, J. (1972). *Play, dreams and imitation.* London: Routledge and Kegan, Paul.

Quilitch, H. R. (1977). The evaluation of children's play material. *Journal of Applied Behavior Analysis, 10*(3), 501-502.

Redl, F. (1972). *When we deal with children.* New York: Free Press.

Rehmann, A., & Riggen, T. (Eds.) (1977). *The least restrictive alternative.* Minneapolis: University of Minnesota Press.

Rinn, R., & Markle, A. (1979). Modification of skills deficits in children. In A. Bellack & M. Hersen (Eds.), *Research and practice in social skills training.* New York: Plenum.

Roff, M., Sells, B., & Golden, N. (1972). *Social adjustment and personality development in children.* Minneapolis: University of Minnesota Press.

Ross, A. L., & Bernstein, N. D. (1976). A framework for the therapeutic use of group activities. *Child Welfare, 55*(9), 627-640.

Rumanoff, L. N. (1978). Developing group names for children with severe learning and behavior disorders. *Teaching Exceptional Children, 10,* 51-53.

Rushakoff, G., & Lombardino, L. (1983). Comprehensive microcomputer applications for severely physically handicapped children. *Teaching exceptional children.*

Sabatino, D., & Schloss, P. (1981). Adolescent social-personal development: Theory and application. In D. Sabatino, C. Schmdt, & T. Miller (Eds.), *Learning disabilities: Systemizing, teaching and service delivery.* Rockville, MD: Aspen Publications.

Sailor, W., & Haring, N. (1977). Some current directions in education of the severely/multiply handicapped. *AAESPH Review, 2,* 68-87.

Salend, S. J. (1981). Cooperative games promote positive student interactions. *Teaching Exceptional Children, 13*(2), 76-80.

Schloss, P. (1984). *Social development of handicapped children and adolescents.* Rockville, MD: Aspen Publications.

Sherrill, C. (1976). *Adapted physical education and recreation: A multidisciplinary approach.* Dubuque, IA: W. C. Brown.

Sirvis, B., & Cieloha, D. (1981). Recreation and leisure skills. In J. Umbreit & P. Cardullias (Eds.), *Educating the severely physically handicapped: Curriculum adaptations, 4,* 53-64, Columbus, OH: Special Press.

Spitz, R. (1972). Fundamental education. In W. Piers (Ed.), *Play and development.* New York: Norton.

Strain, P. (1975). Increasing social play of severely retarded preschoolers. *Mental Retardation, 13*(6), 7-9.

Strain, P. (1982). *Social development of exceptional children.* Rockville, MD: Aspen Publications.

Turner, A. S., Hersen, M., & Bellack, A. S. (1978). Social skills training to teach prosocial behaviors in an organically impaired and retarded patient. *Journal of Behavior Therapy and Experimental Psychiatry, 9*, 253-258.

Wambold, C., & Bailey, R. (1979). Improving the leisure-time behaviors of severely/profoundly mentally retarded children through play. *AAESPH review, 4*, 237-250.

Wehman, P. (1977). *Helping the mentally retarded acquire play skills: A behavioral approach.* Springfield, IL: Charles Thomas Publishing Co.

Wehman, P. (1979). Instructional strategies for improving toy play skills of severely handicapped children. *AAESPH review, 4*, 125-135.

Wehman, P., & Marchant, J. (1978). Improving free play skills of severely retarded children. *American Journal of Occupational Therapy, 32*, 100-104.

Wehman, P., & Schleien, S. J. (1981). *Leisure programs for handicapped persons.* Baltimore: University Park Press.

Whitehill, M., Hersen, M., & Bellack, A. (1980). Conversation skills training for socially isolated children. *Behavior Research and Theory, 18*, 217-225.

Wickersham, C., & Bland, L. (1977). *Behavioral characteristics progression.* Palo Alto, CA: VORT Corp., 1977.

Research and Trends in Employment of Adolescents with Handicaps

John S. Trach
Frank R. Rusch

ABSTRACT. This paper focuses on current, curriculum programming trends that appear to be facilitating the transition of adolescents with handicaps into "everyday" community settings. Traditional curriculum models have failed to enhance or improve attainment of integration into the community; recent attempts to focus curriculum outcomes on the adult life or community-referenced curriculum models appear more promising. Similarly, traditional instructional strategies appear to only partially prepare students for employment, whereas new curriculum models seem to incorporate strategies, such as self-control, which promote maintenance and generalization. These newer curricular focuses and recent advances in teaching strategies may be key factors that ensure integration and transition into community work settings.

In our public schools, efforts have been directed toward teaching students with handicaps in "everyday" community settings. This

John Trach and Frank Rusch are affiliated with the University of Illinois at Urbana-Champaign, College of Education, 288 Education Building, 1310 S. 6 Street, Champaign, IL 61820. This paper was supported in part by the Office of Special Education and Rehabilitative Services, United States Department of Education pursuant to grant numbers OEG-0082-00415 and OEG 0084-30081. However, the opinions expressed herein do not necessarily reflect the position or policy of the Office of Special Education and Rehabilitative Services, United States Department of Education, nor of the University of Illinois, and no official endorsement should be inferred. Copies can be obtained from either author, Office of Career Development for Special Populations, 345 Education Building, College of Education, 1310 South 6 Street, Champaign, IL 61820. Special thanks are extended to Lizanne DeStefano for her critical reading of an earlier draft.

integration has gone beyond the physical placement of handicapped youth in educational settings with nonhandicapped youth. Programs that create opportunities for interaction between handicapped and nonhandicapped persons across a variety of community settings are becoming increasingly popular (Wilcox & Bellamy, 1982). Recently, the notion of community integration was defined as "the process of uniting handicapped and nonhandicapped individuals as equal members jointly participating in recreational, residential, and employment settings" (Rusch, Chadsey-Rusch, White, & Gifford, 1985, p. 120). To complement and facilitate this trend toward integration, educational goals have begun to focus upon preparing students to function in "a variety of post-secondary vocational, domestic, and community environments" (Wilcox & Bellamy, 1982, p. 6).

Recreational, residential, and employment environments hold equal importance in defining the community and thus are difficult to consider separately when discussing community integration. However, the employment component of the adult life curriculum model as a method of integrating individuals with handicaps into the community work force, serves as the primary focus of this paper (Rusch et al., 1985). We will discuss research and trends in establishing goals for employment outcomes, including the varying instructional methodologies used to attain those goals, in the context of both traditional and community-referenced adult life curriculum models. Because the ultimate goal of transition to community living cannot be dissected from discussion of other points in employment education, the concept of transition is used to integrate and give meaning to these efforts in the education of persons with handicaps for employment. To this end, we will examine the adult life curriculum model and its accompanying instructional strategies with respect to their effectiveness in facilitating transition from secondary school to adult life in the community.

TRANSITION

The transition of the adolescent with handicaps into the world of work and productivity must be a planned endeavor. Transition plans need to be developed when a child first enters school, then continually refined and revised as students progress through their public school experience (Bates, 1984; Brown, Pumpian, Baumgart, Vandeventer, Ford, Nisbet, Schroeder, & Gruenewald, 1981; Rusch & Chadsey-Rusch, in press). At the secondary level, transition planning must be a very active component of the student's program (Wilcox & Bellamy, 1982). Wehman's (1984) definition of vocational transition typifies this trend of carefully planned transition:

> Vocational transition is a carefully planned process, which may be initiated either by school personnel or adult service providers, to establish and implement a plan for either employment or additional vocational training of a handicapped student who will graduate or leave in three to five years; such a process must involve special educators, vocational educators, parents and/or the student, and adult service system representative, and possibly an employer. (p. 2-3)

Will (1984) describes three stages of transition: (a) school instruction, (b) plans for the transition process, and (c) placement into meaningful employment. She describes transition as a "bridge" from the security and structure of high school to the opportunities and risks of adult life, stressing that any bridge must have a strong foundation at either end. Employment should be the outcome of education and transition.

According to the Office of Special Education and Rehabilitative Services (OSERS), the goal of transition is to enable the handicapped person to obtain a job either immediately after leaving school or after a period of post-secondary education or vocational services, regardless of the presence, nature, or severity of a disability. The OSERS transition model contains three levels. The *first* involves movement from school either without services or with only those that are available to the population at large; the *second* involves use of time-limited services that are designed to lead to independent employment at termination of service; and the *third* involves the use of ongoing services for those individuals who do not move to unsupported work roles (Will, 1984). Traditionally, only the first two levels exist as vocational options for individuals with handicaps. The first level accommodates the most mildly handicapped and economically disadvantaged, while the second level accommodates individuals with mild handicaps and a few individuals with moderate handicaps. The majority of individuals with moderate and severe handicaps attend a sheltered workshop. Sheltered workshops have stood in place of the third level of service, occurring more frequently than more contemporary options such as supported work and supported employment.

During secondary education, the focus of transition must first be on developing a strong foundation for the public school's end of the "bridge." Wehman (1984) identified three necessary elements of a secondary special education program: (a) a functional curriculum, (b) an integrated school environment, and (c) community-based service delivery. Through such a program, potential employers will be able to observe the students' competent performance of community jobs (Brown, 1984). The next step in the transition involves active negotiation and coordination with adult service agencies.

Though the importance of carefully planned transition to community life for adolescents with handicaps is obvious, current investigations and discussions of curriculum model development (Brown, 1984; Wehman, 1984; Will, 1984) emphasize the need to address the woeful lack of transition planning.

CURRICULUM MODELS

Several widely used curriculum models for the instruction of students who are handicapped have been developed in recent years. These models can be divided into traditional models and adult life models. Traditional models have a long standing history and vary greatly in their theoretical orientations. The traditional models include (a) the eliminative education model, (b) the developmental education model, and (c) the basic skills or early academic content model. Adult life models are generally community-referenced, emphasizing the handicapped individual's present or future functioning needs in the community. These models consider both transition and integration and have been well represented by Bates (1984; in press); Brown, Branston, Hamre-Nietupski, Pumpian, Certo, and Gruenewald (1979); Rusch (1983); Wehman, Renzaglia, and Bates (1985); and Wilcox and Bellamy (1982).

Traditional Models

The first of the traditional models, the *eliminative education model*, may be more of a process which places greatest emphasis upon the elimination of inappropriate behaviors of persons with handicaps than a comprehensive curriculum model (Barrett, 1979). Historically, individuals with handicaps were labelled and removed from society into segregated facilities (Rusch et al., 1985). The eliminative model advocates such segregation until maladaptive behaviors are reduced to a socially acceptable level. At the secondary level this segregation further delays meaningful instruction. Indeed, in its emphasis on controlling inappropriate behaviors, the eliminative process neglects both the development of appropriate behaviors and community integration outcomes. Consideration of transition and generalization based on anything other than functional skills in the normal environment is reduced to secondary emphasis. Because segregation promotes neither transition to the community nor generalization of skills to community settings, these aims are given secondary emphasis.

The second traditional model, *the developmental education model*, has its roots in developmental theory (Bricker, Bricker, Iacino, & Dennison, 1976; Cohen, Gross, & Haring, 1976; Haring & Bricker, 1976). This model holds that all handicapped children proceed through the same developmental stages that characterize normal development. This developmental sequence is usually broken down into gross motor, fine motor, perceptual, cognitive, social, and self-help domains. There are several serious problems with this model, particularly as children grow and mature into adolescents and adults. The central premise that handicapped children must go through the same developmental sequence as their nonhandicapped peers, but at a much slower pace, lacks empirical support since adolescents with handicaps usually develop differently than their nonhandicapped peers (Brown et al., 1979; Wilcox & Bellamy, 1982). It is also unlikely that development will occur at the same rate across all domains. Wilcox and Bellamy (1982) cite the nonexistence of functional alternatives when a child is incapable of performing the normal requisites of a developmental sequence (i.e., inability to walk). Practically, there is not enough time for an adolescent in a secondary program to progress through the developmental stages he/she may not have mastered. Therefore, strict adherence to developmental sequence in educational planning can result in instructional objectives that are sequenced according to developmental stage learning, and which may be nonfunctional and inappropriate given the student's age and pattern of individual strengths and weaknesses (Certo, 1983; Wehman et al., 1985; Wilcox & Bellamy, 1982). For example, a developmentally-oriented education program for a severely handicapped student may emphasize the development of gross and fine motor skills as prerequisites to development in other domains. As a result, this student may master completion of a formboard or pegboard, but may lack grooming, toileting, and appropriate leisure skills. It is unlikely that the community will accept an 18-year-old student who has limited grooming skills, cannot toilet himself, and plays with Tinkertoys! Thus, the developmental education model may hinder an individual's transition into adult life as a participant in work, leisure, and residential settings, offering instruction appropriate for his developmental stage but leaving him unfamiliar with the social norms of their same-aged peers and sadly unprepared for adult life.

The third traditional model evolves from the *early academic* or *"basic skills" approach*, in which the handicapped child's development in traditional academic areas is compared with that of his nonhandicapped peers. Wilcox and Bellamy (1982) cite three major problems with this approach: (a) the approach burdens the student with the responsibility to integrate the "basic skills" to complex community settings; (b) the emphasis is on the specific skill (e.g., making change or telling time) as opposed to the function of the skills taught (e.g., purchasing items or managing time throughout the day); and (c) there is insufficient time to develop basic academic skills to a level of competent and functional application. Students with handicaps may never progress beyond the prerequisite academic skills. Therefore, this model shares the weakness identified with the developmental model discussed earlier. These problems are sufficient to bar consideration of the early academic model as a viable curriculum strategy because the model does little to actively promote integration and impedes transition into normal community settings.

Adult Life Model

The *adult life model* represents the current trend in curriculum development. The adult life model examines the demands the student will face as an adult and determines the curriculum accordingly, rather than paralleling the curriculum appropriate to the development of nonhandicapped peers. The model is referenced to the student's own community to maximize relevance and individualization. Several such models have been described in the literature (Bates, in press; Brown et al., 1979; Wehman et al., 1985; Wilcox & Bellamy, 1982). These models share the main thrust of integration of the handicapped individual as an actively contributing member of the community. In the same spirit, Bates (in press) prefaces his service delivery model for "Project EARN" with the program philosophy of zero exclusion, integration, and normalization.

The adult life model prescribes the sequence of secondary school preparation for employment presented in Table 1. The first four steps are primarily assessment tasks while steps 5, 6, 7, and 8 address the training functions involved in secondary preparation for employment. Step 1 is an ecological or environmental inventory of potential employment possibilities within the particular individual's community. These inventories reflect jobs that are presently avail-

Table 1

Steps for Secondary Preparation for Employment

Assessment Functions	1.	Identify Available Jobs in the Community
	2.	Assess Job Requisites (Entry Level Skills)
	3.	Establish Work Performance Objectives
	4.	Assess Student Performance and Develop Individualized Education Program.
Training Functions	5.	Teach Students to Perform Entry Level Skills in Community-Based Employment Training Programs
	6.	Place Students in Target Placement
	7.	Teach Students to Perform New Skills and to Maintain Entry Level Skills
	8.	Systematically Withdraw Post-Placement Instruction Program

able in the community where the student will ultimately be an active participant.

Step 2 is a job skill inventory that assesses job requisites and delineates necessary job skills within a job category. Bellmore and Brown (1978) developed a "Job Skill Inventory" to break identified jobs down into instructionally manageable components. Wilcox and Bellamy (1982) proposed the development of a "catalog" to delineate job related activities within domains (vocational, independent living, and leisure) and across environments (home, school, and community). Both methods are geared toward identifying the activities, requisite skills, or survival skills necessary for successful job placement. These skills may not be directly related to a specific job, but may be work related skills (e.g., money, transportation).

Step 3 is a determination of work performance objectives and task analysis which further defines the structure of the curriculum from which instructional choices can be made. Because these choices are value judgments (Wilcox & Bellamy, 1982), they should be socially validated (Rusch, 1983; Wehman et al., 1985). That is, objectives selected from the curriculum must reflect not only student potential and interest, but also employment goals that are both supported by parents and are also available in the community. Thus, Step 4, parent consultation, represents the adult life model's commitment to strong parental and student involvement in selecting job skills to be taught and in developing the student's Individualized Education Program.

Summary

This section introduced several curriculum models that have been the traditional focus of educators as well as a relatively new model, the adult life model. The adult life model suggests that a new approach is needed. This approach is directed toward current and future environments. A distinguishing feature of this model is the process used to establish educational outcomes. The survey-then-validate approach, which enjoins the parent's and the student's expectations, appears unique. The next section of this paper identifies new instructional strategies that warrant consideration by educators as they promote the students' independence and adaptability in current and future settings.

INSTRUCTIONAL STRATEGIES

As community-referenced curricula increase in popularity, more training is now taking place in community-based settings (refer to Table 1, Step 5). The primary rationale for providing instruction in the community is to minimize the differences between training and placement settings, thus eliminating some of the problems of generalization that may limit integration opportunities of persons with handicaps (Brown et al., 1979). Physical integration is attained by teaching individuals with handicaps in settings in which they will live, work, and recreate. Instruction is geared toward achieving integration by active participation, enabling the handicapped individual to maintain a target placement within, for example, the employment setting (Step 6) through performance of clearly specified and trained job skills (Step 7). When these job skills are performed to an acceptable level, effort is made to withdraw instruction in a manner that results in the target behaviors being controlled by natural reinforcers (Step 8).

A new instructional technology, which is tied to the adult life model, has evolved to better address the trend toward integrating handicapped individuals into the work community. In addition to traditional methods of instruction, which are crucial in the acquisition phase of job skill training, this new technology is aimed at the development of autonomy and adaptability, reflecting the transition and integration phases of the adult life model (Gifford, Rusch, Martin, & White, 1984; Rusch, Gifford, & Chadsey-Rusch, 1984). *Autonomy* is based on the acquisition of maintenance skills, or the ability to perform vocational skills with minimal supervision. *Adaptability* is associated with generalization, or the ability to perform vocational skills in nontrained employment settings. Training may differentially emphasize autonomy and adaptability. If the target work setting is known, emphasis should be placed upon the goals of autonomy; in instances where work placements are not known, adaptability should be the focus of instruction, because this approach teaches students to adapt what they have learned to new situations. However, the overriding emphasis of training for all individuals with handicaps should be to maximize both autonomy and adaptability in the work situation.

Traditional Strategies of Instruction

Rusch (1983) and Wehman (1981) have documented that handicapped individuals are capable of acquiring competencies necessary for employment. A common set of instructional methods have been developed. Snell (1982) described these traditional methods of systematic instruction in relation to general education goals. Many of these same procedures (e.g., task analysis, levels of assistance, contingent and social reinforcement, repeated practice) are routinely employed in vocational training and are described in the literature (Bates & Pancsofar, 1981; Bellamy, Horner, & Inman, 1979; Renzaglia, Bates, & Hutchins, 1981; Rusch & Mithaug, 1980; Wehman, 1981; Wilcox & Bellamy, 1982). The traditional instructional methods used in vocational training are generally divided into two groups; those which facilitate acquisition of job skills, and those which increase productivity (Brown & Pearce, 1970; Cuvo, Leaf, & Borakove, 1978; Gold, 1972; Martin, Pallotta-Cornick, Johnstone, & Goyos, 1980; Renzaglia, Wehman, Schutz, & Karan, 1978; Spooner & Hendrickson, 1976).

Acquisition training usually begins with the development of a task analysis for assessment and teaching (Gold & Pomerantz, 1978; Renzaglia et al., 1981). Arrangement of task materials, devices, or prosthesis for job completion and setting variables must be considered before the actual training of the task. Training is conducted by either backward or forward chaining or simultaneous instruction across all steps in the task (Bellamy et al., 1979; Renzaglia et al., 1981). Bellamy et al. (1979) recommended using individual instruction, forward chaining, and simultaneous instruction in combination on all steps to teach a task. Their procedure involves four components of training: (a) step training, (b) teaching difficult steps, (c) chain training, and (d) setting training.

Step training involves teaching each step of the task analysis that the worker does not perform correctly 80% of the time. If the student has difficulty meeting this criterion with standard instruction, then *difficult steps training* is used for more intensive training or job modification, once again aimed at attaining the 80% criterion. These first two steps involve more intensive and consistent reinforcement and assistance than chain training. *Chain training* involves teaching larger units of behavior through the use of intermittent reinforcement and assistance. This training utilizes standard training techniques such as levels of assistance, graduated guidance, and prompting (Bates & Pancsofar, 1981; Bellamy et al., 1979; Renzaglia et al., 1981; Rusch & Mithaug, 1980; Snell, 1982; Wilcox & Bellamy, 1982).

The fourth stage of the Bellamy et al. (1979) training model is referred to as *setting training*. At this level the student has already learned the task in an instructional situation and must now perform it under the more natural contingencies of the work environment. Bates (in press), Wehman et al. (1985), and Wilcox and Bellamy (1982) all point to the necessity of bringing appropriate behaviors for employment and community living under the direct control of natural contingencies. Wehman et al. (1985) caution teaching student dependence on the teacher, which is usually established during acquisition training. Traditionally, Steps 5, 7, and 8 in Table 1 utilize these strategies to gradually move the student toward independence.

New Focus for Instruction: Autonomy and Adaptability

A new focus for instruction has been presented in a recent series of articles (Gifford et al., 1984; Rusch et al., 1984; Rusch et al., 1985), that describe the need to focus upon independence and adaptability. By using the terms "autonomy" and "adaptability," instead of maintenance and generalization, this literature now empowers the individual with these attributes rather than recognizing them as a general outcome.

Training toward *autonomy* involves the use of (a) traditional instructional strategies, (b) self-control strategies, and (c) withdrawal design strategies. *Traditional instructional strategies* have already been discussed. They include training in community-based settings in order to minimize differences in skill requisites and setting, as well as arrangement of task materials and devices to aid in completion of a task. *Self-control strategies* teach the individual to regulate his or her own behavior. Antecedent cue regulation, such as using picture cues, is one type of self-control strategy that has shown much promise (Martin, Rusch, James, Decker, & Intol, 1982; Robinson-Wison, 1977; Spellman, DeBrieve, Jarboe, Campbell, & Harris, 1978). Other common strategies are self-monitoring and self-instruction of behavior (Wehman, Schutz, Bates, Renzaglia, & Karan, 1978; Zohn & Bornstein, 1980). *Withdrawal designs* consist of systematically withdrawing training components, such as cues or reinforcement, and monitoring the independence of the student (Martin et al., 1982; Vogelsberg & Rusch, 1979). Assessing the withdrawal of teaching strategies relates to Step 8 which results in leaving intact the gains of the teaching process, yet withdrawing all extraneous variables. Three withdrawal designs include (a) the sequential-withdrawal design, which consists of withdrawing selected components of instructional packages in consecutive phases of teaching; (b) the partial-withdrawal design, which consists of withdrawing part or all of the package for one or several different behaviors, persons, or settings; and (c) the partial-sequential withdrawal design, which consists of a combination of the two previous withdrawal strategies (Gifford et al., 1984; Rusch et al., 1984; Rusch & Kazdin, 1981). The two most important features of the withdrawal designs are that (a) the target behavior is maintained through assessment while the teacher withdraws instructional programs from the training situations, and that (b) the student learns to maintain appropriate behavior in the target work setting using only naturally occurring contingencies.

Adaptability is usually associated with general-case programming (Gifford et al., 1984). Horner, Sprague, and Wilcox (1982, p. 63) define general-case programming as "those behaviors performed by the teacher or trainer that increase the probability that skills learned in one training setting will be successfully performed with different target stimuli and/or in different settings from those used during training." In other words, the teacher must select appropriate examples representative of the instructional universe (e.g., selective work setting) and train those examples in a sequence that promotes generalization.

Two key concepts in this process are *stimulus class* and *response class. Stimulus class* refers to any group of stimuli that share a common set of stimulus characteristics. To be a member, the stimulus must have all the relevant characteristics of the class. For example, members of the stimulus class, nails, would all possess a common set of attributes (i.e., metal, flat head, smooth shaft, point). All stimuli that do not have those attributes (e.g., screws) would be outside this class. A *response class* is a set of behaviors that produce the same functional outcome. A general case is learned when any instance from a stimulus class prompts the student to demonstrate the appropriate member of a response class. For example, presentation of a member of the stimulus class, nails, prompts the student to select and appropriately use a hammer to pound a nail into a piece of wood. Trained and untrained instances of a stimulus class control trained and untrained members of a response class (Horner et al., 1982, p. 67). General case programming increases the probability of generalized responding (Horner & McDonald, 1982; Rusch et al., 1985; Sprague & Horner, 1984).

Rusch et al., (1984) found a paucity of research focusing upon both autonomy and adaptability. In order to attain both transition and integration of adolescents with handicaps, teachers and researchers must attend to the need for students to perform job skills in natural settings with minimal supervision, and to perform tasks across environmental contexts that are different from those in which instruction took place. Integration cannot take place if the presence of the teacher is required to ensure appropriate behavior, or if the target individual is restricted to certain settings or conditions because of situation-specific instructional outcomes.

Summary

The literature on autonomy and adaptability provides new directions for instruction by assigning certain instructional attributes (i.e., autonomy and adaptability) to the individual rather than to the instructional process. Nevertheless, only Wacker and Berg (1983) addressed both concepts of autonomy and adaptability in one study. There is an obvious need for more research and development in this area. For integration to go beyond physical placement toward independence, and for transition to adult life to be realized, the individual must be more autonomous and adaptable. Acceptance by the community will be judged by demonstration of competence that more closely approximates the expectations of how an active participant of that community functions.

GENERAL SUMMARY

This review concentrated on current trends in employment education of adolescents with handicaps. The main focus was realizing the goals of transition and integration into adult life. The current trend of the community-referenced curriculum and community-based instruction attains physical integration, but does not assure a level of independence (autonomy) or performance (adaptability) that may enhance long-term placement in natural settings. Transition becomes more attainable using adult-life curriculum models to minimize the differences between training environments and expected employment environments for performance of learned skills. Both transition and integration are evaluated in reference to the concept of normalization. Normalization is based on the premise that people must learn skills that enhance community acceptance (Nirje, 1969; Wolfensberger, 1972). The key to acceptance will be the performance of the learned skills in the community.

The adult life model discussed addresses transition to adult life and suggests some methods of attaining this goal. However, there is a dearth of instruction that focuses on integration. Acquisition strategies are of limited value. Maintenance and generalization must be considered in the same systematic fashion as acquisition training. At this time, maintenance and generalization outcomes have received little attention in the employment literature (Horner et al., 1982; Rusch, Martin, & White, in press).

One could conclude from this review that many models of preparation of adolescents with handicaps for employment claim to facilitate transition and integration. With the exception of Step 8, Table 1 is such a model. The first four steps describe a community-referenced, adult-life curriculum model. Step 5 maximizes transfer and generalization of training (i.e., one's adaptability). Step 6 plans for transition by placing the student in the job he/she would have after graduation, and Step 7 adjusts the training to the new job setting. At this point, unless general case programming is overlaid on Steps 5 and 7, adaptability is limited. Likewise, unless training for autonomy is developed in Step 4 and finalized in Step 8 the individual's integration and transition into adult life my remain at the physical level. Steps 6, 7, and 8 emphasize transition as a concept that must be programmed at the secondary level.

Implementation of the adult-life model and future research activities focusing upon autonomy and adaptability should improve the transition process. Autonomy and adaptability appear to be key factors ensuring adolescents a meaningful place in integrated employment settings. Indeed, instruction should facilitate one's independence and freedom from supervision for all individuals with handicaps.

REFERENCES

Barrett, B. (1979). Communitization and the measured message of normal behavior. In R. York & E. Edgar (Eds.), *Teaching the severely handicapped, Vol. 4.* Columbus, OH: Special Press.

Bates, P. (1984). *Vocational curriculum development for persons labeled mentally retarded.* Paper presented at the National Symposium on Employment of Citizens with Mental Retardation, Rehabilitation Research and Training Center, Virginia Commonwealth University, Virginia Beach.

Bates, P. (in press). Project EARN (Employment and rehabilitation = normalization): A service delivery model for enhancing competitive employment outcomes for moderately and severely handicapped youth in the public schools. In F. R. Rusch (Ed.), *Competitive employment: Service delivery models, methods, and issues.* Baltimore: Paul H. Brookes.

Bates, P. & Pancsofar, E. (1981). Longitudinal vocational training for severely handicapped students in the public schools. In R. York, W. K. Schofield, D. J. Donder, D. L. Ryndak, & B. Reguly (Eds.), *Proceedings from the 1981 Illinois Statewide Institute for Educators of the Severely and Profoundly Handicapped.* Springfield, IL: Department of Specialized Educational Services, Illinois Board of Education.

Bellamy, G. T., Horner, R., & Inman, D. (1979). *Vocational training of severely retarded adults.* Baltimore: University Park Press.

Belmore, K. & Brown, L. (1978). Job skill inventory strategy for use in a public school vocational training program for severely handicapped potential workers. In N. Haring & D. Bricker (Eds.), *Teaching the severely handicapped, Vol. III.* Columbus, OH: Special Press.

Bricker, D., Bricker, W., Iacino, R., & Dennison, L. (1976). Intervention strategies for the severely and profoundly handicapped child. In N. J. Haring & L. J.

Brown (Eds.), *Teaching the severely handicapped, Vol. 1.* New York: Grune & Stratton.

Brown, J. M. (1984). A model for enhancing the transition of mildly handicapped youth into post-secondary vocational education. In J. Chadsey-Rusch (Ed.), *Conference Proceedings from "Enhancing Transition from School to the Workplace for Handicapped Youth. "* Urbana-Champaign, IL: Office of Career Development for Special Populations, University of Illinois.

Brown, L., Branston, M., Hamre-Nietupski, S., Pumpian, I., Certo, N., & Gruenewald, L. (1979). A strategy for developing chronological age-appropriate and functional curricular content for severely handicapped adolescents and young adults. *Journal of Special Education, 13,* 81-9.

Brown, L. & Pearce, E. (1970). Increasing the production rates of trainable retarded students in a public school simulated workshop. *Education and Training of the Mentally Retarded, 5,* 15-22.

Brown, L., Pumpian, I., Baumgart, D., Vandeventer, P., Ford, A., Nisbet, J., Schroeder, J., & Gruenewald, L. (1981). Longitudinal transition plans in programs for severely handicapped students. *Exceptional Children, 47,* 624-631.

Certo, N. (1983). Characteristics of educational services. In M. Snell (Ed.), *Systematic instruction of the moderately and severely handicapped* (2nd ed.). Columbus, OH: Charles E. Merrill.

Cohen, M., Gross, P., & Haring, N. G. (1976). Developmental pinpoints. In N. H. Haring & L. M. Brown (Eds.), *Teaching the severely handicapped, Vol. 1.* New York: Grune & Stratton.

Cuvo, A., Leaf, R., & Borakove, L. (1978). Teaching janitorial skills to the mentally retarded: Acquisition, generalization, and maintenance. *Journal of Applied Behavior Analysis, 11,* 345-355.

Gifford, J. L., Rusch, F. R., Martin, F. R., & White, D. M. (1984). Autonomy and adaptability in work behavior of retarded clients. In N. R. Ellis & N. W. Bray (Eds.), *International Review of Research in Mental Retardation, Vol. 12.* New York: Academic Press.

Gold, M. (1972). Stimulus factors in skill training of the retarded on a complex assembly task: Acquisition, transfer, and retention. *American Journal of Mental Deficiency, 76,* 517-526.

Gold, M. & Pomerantz, D. (1978). Issues in prevocational training. In M. Snell (Ed.), *Systematic instruction of the moderately and severely handicapped.* Columbus, OH: Charles E. Merrill.

Haring, N. G. & Bricker, D. (1976). Overview of comprehensive services for the severely/profoundly handicapped. In N. H. Haring & L. J. Brown (Eds.), *Teaching the severely handicapped, Vol. 1.* New York: Grune & Stratton.

Horner, R. H. & McDonald, R. S. (1982). A comparison of single instance and general case instruction in teaching a generalized vocational skill. *The Journal of the Association for the Severely Handicapped, 7,* 7-20.

Horner, R. H., Sprague, J., & Wilcox, B. (1982). General case programming for community activities. In B. Wilcox & G. T. Bellamy (Eds.), *Design of high school programs for severely handicapped students*, Baltimore: Paul H. Brookes.

Martin, G., Pallotta-Cornick, A., Johnstone, G., & Goyos, A. (1980). A supervisory strategy to improve work performance for lower functioning retarded clients in a sheltered workshop. *Journal of Applied Behavior Analysis, 13*, 183-190.

Martin, J. E., Rusch, R. R., James, V. L., Decker, P. J., & Trtol, K. A. (1982). The use of picture cues to establish self-control in the preparation of complex meals by mentally retarded adults. *Applied Research in Mental Retardation, 3*, 105-119.

Nirje, B. (1968). The normalization principle and its human management implications. In R. Kugel & W. Wolfensberger (Eds.), *Changing patterns of residential services for the mentally retarded*. Washington, DC: President's Committee on Mental Retardation.

Renzaglia, A., Bates, P., & Hutchins, M. (1981). Vocational skills instruction for handicapped adolescents and adolescents and adults. *Exceptional Education Quarterly, 2*, 61-73.

Renzaglia, A., Wehman, P., Schutz, R., & Karan, O. (1978). Use of cue redundancy and positive reinforcement to accelerate production in two profoundly retarded workers. *British Journal of Social and Clinical Psychology, 17*, 183-187.

Robinson-Wilson, M. (1977). Picture recipe cards as an approach to teaching severely and profoundly retarded adults to cook. *Education and Training of the Mentally Retarded, 12*, 69-73.

Rusch, F. R. (1983). Competitive vocational training. In M. Snell (Ed.), *Systematic instruction of the moderately and severely handicapped* (2nd ed.). Columbus, OH: Charles E. Merrill.

Rusch, F. R., Chadsey-Rusch, J., White, D. M., & Gifford, J. L. (1985). Programs for severely mentally retarded adults: Perspectives and methodologies. In D. Bricker & J. Filler (Eds.), *The severely mentally retarded: From research to practice*. Reston, VA: Council for Exceptional Children.

Rusch, F. R. & Chadsey-Rusch, U. (in press). Employment for persons with severe handicaps: Curriculum development and coordination of services. *Focus on Exceptional Children*.

Rusch, F. R. Gifford, J. L., & Chadsey-Rusch, J. (1984). *Behavioral training strategies and applied research in competitive employment*. Paper presented at the National Symposium on Employment of Citizens With Mental Retardation. Rehabilitation Research and Training Center, Virginia Commonwealth University, Virginia Beach.

Rusch, F. R. & Kazdin, A. E. (1981). Toward a methodology of withdrawal designs for the assessment of response maintenance. *Journal of Applied Behavior Analysis, 14*, 131-140.

Rusch, F. R., Martin, J. E., & White, D. M. (in press). Competitive employment: Teaching mentally retarded employees to maintain their work behavior. *Mental Retardation*.

Rusch, F. R., & Mithaug, D. E. (1980). *Vocational training for mentally retarded adults*. Champaign, IL: Research Press.

Snell, M. (Ed.) (1982). *Systematic instruction of the moderately and severely handicapped*. Columbus, OH: Charles E. Merrill.

Spellman, C., DeBriere, T., Jarboe, D., Campbell, S., & Harris, C. (1978). Pictorial instruction: Training daily living skills. In M. Snell (Ed.), *Systematic instruction of the moderately and severely handicapped*, Columbus, OH: Charles E. Merrill.

Spooner, F. & Hendrickson, B. (1976). Acquisition of complex assembly skills through use of systematic training procedures: Involving profoundly retarded adults. *AAESPH Review, 1*, 14-25.

Sprague, J. & Horner, R. H. (1984). An experimental analysis of generalized vending machine use with severely handicapped students. *Journal of Applied Behavioral Analysis, 17*(2), 273-278.

Vogelsberg, R. T. & Rusch, F. R. (1979). Training severely handicapped students to cross partially controlled intersections. *AAESPH Review, 4*, 264-273.

Wacker, D. & Berg, W. (1983). Effects of picture prompts on the acquisition of complex vocational tasks by mentally retarded adolescents. *Journal of Applied Behavior Analysis, 16*, 417-433.

Wehman, P. (1981). *Competitive employment: New horizons for severely disabled individuals*. Baltimore: Paul H. Brookes.

Wehman, P. (1984). Transition for handicapped youth from school to work. In J. Chadsey-Rusch (Ed.), *Conference Proceedings from "Enhancing Transition from School to the Workplace for Handicapped Youth."* Urbana-Champaign, IL: Office of Career Development for Special Populations, University of Illinois.

Wehman, P., Renzaglia, A., & Bates, P. (1985). *Functional living skills for moderately and severely handicapped individuals*. Austin, TX: Pro-Ed.

Wehman, P., Schutz, R., Bates, P., Renzaglia, A., & Karan, O. (1978). Self-management programs with mentally retarded workers: Implications for developing independent vocational behavior. *British Journal of Social and Clinical Psychology, 17*, 57-64.

Wilcox, B. & Bellamy, G. T. (1982). *Design of high school programs for severely handicapped students*. Baltimore: Paul H. Brookes.

Will, M. (1984). OSERS programming for the transition of youth with disabilities: Bridges from school to working life. In J. Chadsey-Rusch (Ed.), *Conference Proceedings from "Enhancing Transition from School to the Workplace for Handicapped Youth."* Urbana-Champaign, IL: Office of Career Development for Special Populations, University of Illinois.

Wolfensberger, W. (1972). *Principles of normalization*. Toronto: National Institute of Mental Retardation.

Zohn, C. & Bornstein, P. (1980). Self-monitoring of work performance with mentally retarded adults: Effects upon work productivity, work quality, and on-task behavior. *Mental Retardation, 18*, 19-25.

Index